WV577 £25.00
1990

Electric response audiometry in clinical practice

To Jacob Abramovich
Otolaryngologist

Electric response audiometry in clinical practice

Solomon Abramovich MSc FRCS
Consultant Ear, Nose and Throat Surgeon,
St Mary's Hospital and The Central Middlesex Hospital;
Honorary Clinical Senior Lecturer,
Imperial College of Science, Technology and Medicine,
London,
UK

With contributions by

A. R. D. Thornton BSc PhD CEng MBCS MIEE
Scientist in Charge,
MRC Institute of Hearing Research,
Royal South Hants Hospital;
Honorary Reader ISVR,
Southampton University;
Honorary Head of Audiological Sciences,
Royal South Hants Hospital,
Southampton;
Honorary Research Fellow,
Wessex Neurological Centre,
UK

Foreword by

J. L.W. Wright RD FRCS
Consultant Ear, Nose and Throat Surgeon
and Clinical Director,
St Mary's Hospital, London, UK;
Civilian Consultant in Ear, Nose and Throat
Surgery to the Royal Navy;
Consultant in Ear, Nose and Throat Surgery
to the Gibraltar Government

CHURCHILL LIVINGSTONE
EDINBURGH LONDON MELBOURNE AND NEW YORK 1990

CHURCHILL LIVINGSTONE
Medical Division of Longman Group UK Limited

Distributed in the United States of America by Churchill
Livingstone Inc., 1560 Broadway, New York, N.Y. 10036,
and by associated companies, branches and representatives
throughout the world.

First published 1990

ISBN 0-443-03884-8

British Library Cataloguing in Publication Data
Abramovich, Solomon
    Electric-response audiometry in clinical practice.
    1. Man. Hearing disorders. Diagnosis. Electric response
    audiometry
    I. Title   II. Thornton, A. R. D.
    617.8'07544

Library of Congress Cataloging in Publication Data
Abramovich, Solomon.
    Electric-response audiometry in clinical practice/Solomon
    Abramovich, with contributions by A. R. D. Thornton; foreword by
    J. L. W. Wright.
        p. cm.
    Includes bibliographical references.
    ISBN 0-443-03884-8
    1. Audiometry, Evoked response.   I. Thornton, A. R. D.
    II. Title.
        [DNLM: 1. Audiometry, Evoked Response.   WV 272 A242e]
    RF294.5.E87A27   1990
    617.8'07547—dc20
    DNLM/DLC
    for Library of Congress   89–25376
                                                            CIP

Produced by Longman Singapore Publishers (Pte) Ltd.
Printed in Singapore.

Foreword

The measurement of electrical responses to sound stimuli in the auditory system has been increasingly refined during the past three decades, and electric response audiometry has become a familiar diagnostic aid to those professionals working in the field of hearing impairment. Sophisticated techniques are now available to evaluate responses at all anatomical levels in the auditory system. The clinician who has to diagnose and treat those patients unable or unwilling to respond subjectively to routine audiometric tests can now objectively assess the auditory system using the techniques encompassed within the term 'electric response audiometry'. This is particularly pertinent to the detection of early hearing loss in children. Recent advances in surgical treatment of the profoundly deaf by the introduction of the multichannel cochlear implant have highlighted the importance of prior detailed knowledge of the electrophysiologic response in the auditory system of the patient undergoing implantation.

In this comprehensive and authoritative volume, the authors have provided both a reference work and a manual which will find a place in the armamentarium of every practising otologist, audiological physician, and other specialist concerned with the diagnosis and treatment of deafness.

It gives me particular pleasure that this book should, in part, emanate from St Mary's Hospital, which, in 1851, was the first general hospital to designate beds for the treatment of ear disease.

J. L. W. Wright

Preface

Stimulus-related events occurring in the cochlea and auditory pathway exist as bio-electrical potentials which may be recorded from the promontory of the middle ear and the scalp. These electrical responses to a stimulus are known as auditory evoked potentials. They are classified nowadays, according to their latency, into early (0–10 ms), middle (10–50 ms), and late (>50 ms) responses.

The development of electrophysiologic techniques and computer signal-processing has enabled many clinical tests to be based upon these potentials under the name of electric response audiometry (ERA). This has become a useful and objective clinical method in the assessment of auditory dysfunction, being used to estimate auditory thresholds in infants, difficult-to-test children, and other subjects in whom reliability of behavioural audiometric tests is doubtful. It also has a wide range of application in neuro-otological diagnosis.

Although there are now many publications on evoked potentials, these are not always in the most suitable format for the practising otologist and audiologist. The purpose of this book is to provide the otologist with the practical information necessary for application of these tests and to point out the pitfalls in testing and interpretation. The pertinent problems for the clinician are addressed, including the validity of each evoked potential test, its specific application, and appropriate technique.

S. Abramovich.

Abbreviations

ABLB	alternate binaural loudness balance test
ABR	auditory brainstorm response
AC	alternating current
ADC	analogue-to-digital converter
AP	action potential
AVCN	anterior ventral cochlear nucleus
BM	basilar membrane
CAP	compound action potential
CF	characteristic frequency
CM	Cochlear microphonic
CMRR	common-mode rejection ratio
CNS	Central nervous system
CNV	contingent negative variation
CP	cerebello-pontine
CT	computerized tomography
dBA	decibel weighted by the 'A' scale to approximate this physical measurement to the changes in the ear's sensitivity with frequency
dBnHL	decibel threshold at normal hearing level
dBpeSPL	decibel peak equivalent sound pressure level
DC	direct current
DCN	dorsal cochlear nucleus
EABR	Electrically evoked auditory brainstem response
ECochG	electrocochleography
EEG	electroencephalogram
EMLR	electrically evoked middle latency response
ENT	ear, nose, and throat
EP	evoked potential
ERA	electric response audiometry
FFP7	far-field potential 7 (7 ms)
FFR	frequency following response
FTC	frequency tuning curve
HL	hearing level
HTL	hearing threshold level

I-VII	ABR peaks
IAM	internal auditory meatus
ICU	intensive care unit
IHC	inner hair cells
I/O	input/output function
IPI	inter-peak interval
IPL	inter-peak latency
IT 5	interaural latency differential of wave V
LSO	lateral nucleus of superior olive
LV	absolute latency of wave V
MLR	middle latency response
MRI	magnetic resonance imaging
MS	multiple sclerosis
MSO	medial nucleus of superior olive
MTB	medial nucleus of trapezoid body
N	negative polarity peaks
N1, N2, etc.	negative peaks of VIIIth cranial nerve AP
Na, Nb, etc.	negative peaks of middle latency responses
NAP	narrow-band action potential
NOHL	non-organic hearing loss
OHC	outer hair cells
P	positive polarity peaks
P300 (or P3)	late positive component (300 ms)
Pa, Pb, etc.	positive peaks of middle latency responses
PAM	postauricular muscle response
PSP	Postsynaptic potential
PVCN	posterior ventral cochlear nucleus
R–C	rarefaction–condensation
rms	root–mean–square
SCP	sustained cortical potential
SEP	somatosensory-evoked potential
SISI	short increment sensitivity index
SLM	sound level meter
S/N	signal-to-noise ratio
SN10	slow negative wave (10 ms)
SP	summating potential
SPL	sound pressure level
SQUID	superconducting quantum interference device
ST	scala tympani
STIM	stimulus
SV	scala vestibuli
SVR	slow vertex response
TWV	travelling wave velocity
VEP	visual evoked potential
WHO	World Health Organization

Contents

Introduction: Basis of the auditory evoked potentials

1. Historical development of electric response audiometry (ERA)

Spontaneous electrical activity from the scalp was first recorded by Berger in 1929, and this activity is now routinely recorded in the electroencephalogram (EEG). In trying to find electrical activity from the inner ear, Wever & Bray (1930) successfully recorded potentials from the round window of a cat in response to sound stimulation. These potentials approximated the acoustic waveform of the sound, and Adrian (1931) suggested that the responses were generated in the cochlea by some form of microphonic action. They have since become known as the cochlear microphonic (CM). In 1935, Fromm et al made recordings from the round window and the promontory in the human ear, and a similar technique during surgery was later referred to by Lempert et al (1947) as electrocochleography.

Studies were also made on alterations in electroencephalographic recordings in response to sound stimuli. Davis et al (1939) noticed consistent changes in the EEG in response to repeated auditory stimulation. These auditory evoked potentials were best recorded from the vertex, and were initially called 'V' potentials. However, the responses were very small and difficult to measure against the ongoing electrical activity of the brain. Particular difficulty was experienced when the stimuli were of low intensity, as the voltage of the EEG was much greater than that of the evoked potentials. It was therefore not possible to utilize this method for estimation of hearing thresholds with the technology available at that time.

The development of averaging computers facilitated more accurate analysis of small bio-electrical signals. Dawson (1951) was the first to describe a summation technique for the detection of small evoked potentials from the ongoing EEG, and it has since become possible to utilize evoked potentials generated within the auditory system as clinical audiometric tests. The technique of recording the action potential of the cochlear nerve from the round window in an anaesthetized patient was described by Ruben et al (1962). Later a transtympanic technique was popularized by Portmann & Aran (1971). In this technique, a 0.1 mm, insulated, needle electrode is passed down the ear canal through the tympanum to rest on the bony promontory. This technique is now known as transtympanic electrocochleography. Recordings have been made also from electrodes placed in the external ear canal (Yoshie et al 1967, 1971), and from non-invasive surface electrodes placed on the ear lobe and the vertex. The latter technique was described by Sohmer & Feinmesser (1967), who later showed that in addition to the cochlear potentials there were some later waves representing the neural discharge from the brainstem (Sohmer & Feinmesser 1973). Working on animals and later recording from the scalps of humans, Jewett et al (1970, 1971), independently, described the origins of the so-called 'far-field' auditory brainstem potentials recorded from the scalp in response to click stimuli. Middle latency neurogenic responses were described by Mendel & Goldstein (1969). However, in this latency response the potentials were first recorded by Geisler (1958). Other potentials generated along the auditory pathway were also identified. Thousands of research papers and studies on the clinical application of auditory-evoked potentials have been published since that time. Further research in developing stimulation and recording methods is required to optimize EP (evoked potential) techniques for clinical practice.

2. Anatomy, physiology, and classification of the generators of auditory evoked potentials

ANATOMY OF THE EAR AND THE AUDITORY PATHWAY

External auditory meatus and the middle ear

The anatomy of the ear is shown in Figure 2.1, and some of its structures will be described in order to clarify their function in transforming acoustic stimuli into mechanical oscillations and in conducting the stimuli through into the inner ear.

The external auditory apparatus consists of the pinna and external ear canal, which is divided into a lateral membrano-cartilaginous part and a medial bony part. The external auditory meatus has a depth of approximately 28 mm and a diameter of approximately 7 mm. However, the

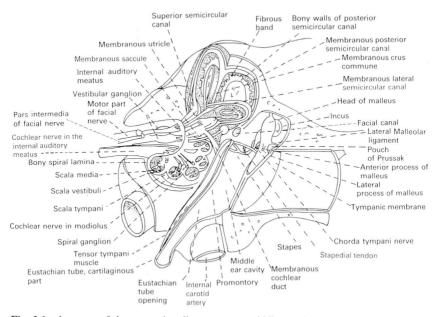

Fig. 2.1 Anatomy of the external auditory meatus, middle ear, inner ear, and internal auditory meatus. (Reproduced with permission from Nicol T & Chao-Charia K K 1981.)

shape of the canal varies to some extent among subjects. Its direction is anteromedial, and the meatus terminates at the tympanic membrane.

The tympanic membrane is approximately 10 mm high and 8 mm long anteroposteriorly, and it resembles the conical diaphragm of a loudspeaker, with a surface area of about 80 mm^2. The larger, vibrating part of the eardrum has a fibrous layer and is called the pars tensa. The smaller, upper portion of the eardrum has little or no fibrous layer and is called the pars flaccida.

The middle-ear cavity is ventilated through the Eustachian tube and contains the articulating ossicles, which are supported by ligaments. The malleus is attached to the tympanic membrane and articulates with the incus. The incus is connected to the head of the stapes, and the footplate of the stapes is, in area, about 3.5 mm^2 and fits into the oval window of the bony labyrinth. The annular ligament surrounds the footplate and allows the stapes to move in the oval window. The tensor tympani muscle is attached to the malleus, and the stapedial muscle to the stapes: these muscles pull in opposite directions and modify the motion of the ossicles. The ossicular chain transmits sound to the cochlea, and the pivotal point of this motion goes through the intermediate ossicle, the body of the incus. The manubrium of the malleus is about 1.3 times longer than the long process of the incus which together can be modelled by a folded lever (Zwislocki 1965).

Cochlea and auditory nerve

As the neuro-anatomy of hearing is extremely complex, only the main anatomical sources pertinent to generation of the different evoked potentials will be mentioned in this chapter. The schematic anatomy of the organ of Corti is shown in Figure 2.2.

The organ of Corti is about 35 mm long and is inside the cochlear duct. It consists of sensory hair cells of 10 μm in diameter and is bounded by the basilar membrane. The sensory cells are surrounded by a variety of supporting cells and by the overlying, gelatinous, tectorial membrane (Fig. 2.2). There is a single row of about 3500 inner hair cells (IHC) and three or four rows of 12 000 outer hair cells (OHC), according to Spoendlin (1986). The outer and inner hair cells are separated by the pillar cells forming the tunnel of Corti, which is filled with the fluid, corticolymph.

Both inner and outer hair cells have the characteristics of mechanoreceptors. The microvilli, or stereocilia, on the surface of the hair cells project towards the tectorial membrane. It is thought that some stereocilia of the outer hair cells are embedded in this membrane. The stereocilia of the same row on each hair cell are joined by horizontally running links. The shorter stereocilia tips also give rise to vertical links, which run upwards to join the taller adjacent stereocilia of the next row (Rhys Evans et al 1985). The movement of the basilar membrane with the endolymph in the cochlear duct

A.

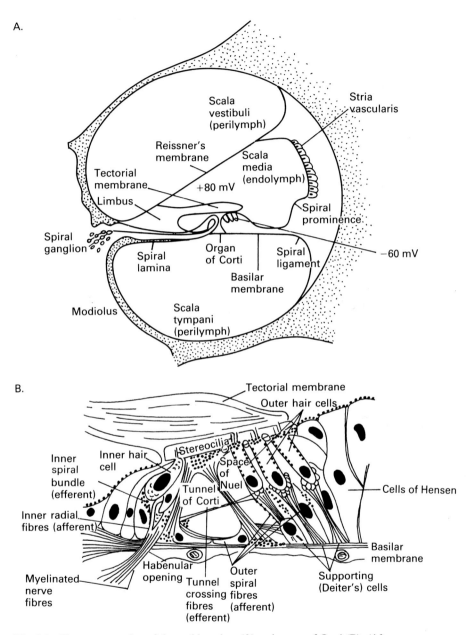

B.

Fig. 2.2 Transverse section of the cochlear duct (**A**) and organ of Corti (**B**). (After (**A**) Pickles J O 1985 and (**B**) Durrant J D & Lovrinic J H 1984, with permission.)

The potentials within the endolymph and the hair cells are shown. This leaves a large potential difference of about 140 mV across the upper surface of the hair cells.

produces the shearing movement of the stereocilia and distortion of the link, a movement which is responsible for bio-electrical transduction.

About 30 000 afferent fibres pass to the hair cells. The cell bodies of the first-order neurones or ganglia are situated in the spiral bony canal in the modiolus. The fibres vary in diameter from 1 to 8 nm, and, as a rule, those connecting to the inner hair cells are thicker than those connecting to the outer hair cells (Gacek & Rasmussen 1961). There is a correlation among fibre size, spontaneous activity, and sensitivity – the thicker fibres being more sensitive and efficient (Liberman 1982). The fibres lose their myelin sheath as they pass into the basilar membrane through small bony canals in the habenula perforata.

About 95% of the afferent neural fibres pass directly to the IHC, while 5% of the afferent fibres cross the tunnel of Corti, mostly in a radial direction, and turn towards the three rows of outer hair cells (see Fig. 2.2). The latter fibres are longer and thinner, and travel towards the basal turn of the cochlea for from one-third to one-fourth of the length of the basilar membrane. It is assumed that they represent a less efficient system than do thicker fibres for transmission of information (Liberman 1982). Thus, it appears that innervation of the outer hair cells is convergent – one neurone communicating with as many as about 10 hair cells – and that innervation of the inner hair cells is divergent – one inner hair cell attaching to many neurones. In general, IHC have a rich afferent nerve supply in contrast to OHC, which have poor afferent innervation and a rich efferent nerve supply (Spoendlin 1986).

The cochlea is innervated by ipsilateral and contralateral efferent fibres. Thin, unmyelinated, efferent fibres make contact with the afferent fibres of the IHC. About 500 efferent fibres of the contralateral olivocochlear bundle cross the tunnel of Corti. They are thought to innervate the outer hair cells and to have a presynaptic inhibitory effect. The good efferent supply and poor afferent system of the OHC suggest that they have an important role at the receptor level, and that the main information transfer relies on the inner hair system and its more efficient afferent pathways (Spoendlin 1986).

Auditory pathway

In this chapter, the afferent auditory pathway is outlined so that its anatomy can be associated with the electrophysiology and generation of evoked potentials in different parts of brain. This pathway is shown schematically in Figure 2.3, which is based on descriptions and reviews by Stelmasiak (1954), Galambos (1958), Crosby and Humphrey (1962), Moller (1983), and Harrison (1987).

The fibres of the first-order neurones originating from the ganglia form the cochlear nerve and enter the brainstem in the upper medulla, terminating in the second-order neurones of the dorsal cochlear nucleus (DCN) or of the anterior and posterior ventral cochlear nucleus (AVCN and PVCN)

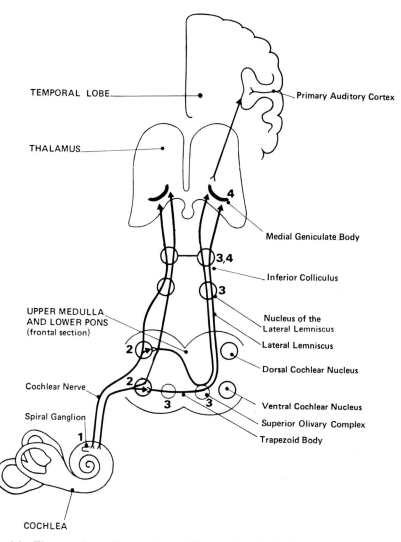

TEMPORAL LOBE

Primary Auditory Cortex

THALAMUS

Medial Geniculate Body

Inferior Colliculus

UPPER MEDULLA
AND LOWER PONS
(frontal section)

Nucleus of the
Lateral Lemniscus

Lateral Lemniscus

Dorsal Cochlear Nucleus

Cochlear Nerve

Spiral Ganglion

Ventral Cochlear Nucleus

Superior Olivary Complex

Trapezoid Body

COCHLEA

Fig. 2.3 The ascending auditory pathways. The numbers 1–4 indicate the order of the neurones.

on the same side. These primary acoustic nuclei constitute neuro-anatomically separate areas and have been fully described by Lorente de No' (1981).

The fibres originating in the ventral cochlear nucleus form synapses with the third-order neurones on both sides in the subnuclei of the superior olivary complex situated in the pontomedullary level. Those fibres from both sides cross over in the ventral stria of the trapezoid body. Fibres from the dorsal cochlear nucleus also cross over, in the dorsal stria of Monakov. In this way, the superior olivary complex, consisting of the lateral nucleus of the superior olive (LSO), the medial nucleus of the superior olive (MSO), and the medial nucleus of the trapezoid body (MTB), receives and relays input from both ears.

Both crossed and uncrossed fibres arising from the cochlear nucleus do not necessarily terminate in the superior olivary complex, but, instead, they may go directly to the inferior colliculus, or they may terminate in the nucleus of the lateral lemniscus.

Most of the third-order neurones from the superior olivary complex pass through the lateral lemniscus, relaying input from the opposite ear, and terminating in the neurones in the inferior colliculus. From there they relay input to the medial geniculate body in the thalamus. There are also interconnections between the two sides at the level of the inferior colliculi. Collaterals from the brainstem auditory pathway go to the reticular formation and the cerebellum.

From the geniculate body the fibres of the fourth-order neurones pass through the acoustic radiation into the tonotopically arranged primary auditory cortex in the temporal lobe. The areas surrounding the primary auditory cortex also participate in auditory function; they are known as secondary and associated auditory areas.

There are also descending corticocochlear efferent pathways, the most peripheral of which are connections to the cochlea from the well-formed crossed and uncrossed fibres from the olivocochlear bundle of Rasmussen (1942), Ward (1978).

BASIC PHYSIOLOGY OF THE AUDITORY SYSTEM

Sound transmission

The outer and the middle ears have an influence on the sound spectrum reaching the ear, and the normal ear in man tends to be most effective in transmitting the frequencies between 2000 and 3000 Hz at low-stimulus intensities (Dallos 1976).

Sound reaching the tympanic membrane sets both it and the ossicular chain vibrating, a vibration, which, in turn, causes a displacement of the stapes in the oval window. This mechanism in the middle ear is responsible for the sound pressure vibrations arriving at the oval window, prior to reaching the round window, and causing a displacement of the basilar membrane.

The role of the external and middle ears is to improve the impedance match between air and the higher impedance of the fluid medium in the cochlea (Tonndorf & Khanna 1976). In the external ear, there is amplification due to the shape of the pinna, diffraction around the head and auricle, and the resonance of the ear canal, all of which combine to give a maximum gain of 20 dB at 3000 Hz (Tonndorf & Khanna 1976). In the middle ear, the major anatomical factor is that the ratio of the large effective area of the tympanic membrane to the small area of the footplate of the stapes is about 18.6. This means that the sound pressure is amplified 18.6

times. Additional amplification of about 1.3 times is caused by the leverage effect of the ossicles; all together, the sound pressure is amplified by about 24 times (1.3 × 18.6) (Zwislocki 1965, 1975). However, one should bear in mind that the sound pressure transmission is effective only if there is sufficiently rapid vibration of the stapes. The mechanical transmission of the middle ear causes a displacement of the basilar membrane, leading to mechano-electrical effects which generate the cochlear microphonic (CM). The CM magnitude, in the basal turn of the cochlea, is largely determined by the middle-ear transmission and by the velocity of the movement of the stapes (Dallos 1976).

Any change in one of the determiners of middle-ear function, such as elasticity, friction, or mass, can lead to a change in the impedance, and can subsequently alter the efficiency of energy transfer. An important physiologic increase in middle-ear impedance occurs at high-stimulus intensities of about 80 dBnHL, when the stapedial muscle reflexively contracts bilaterally, causing some stiffening of the ossicular chain. This is called the acoustic stapedial reflex, and it can be recorded with the impedance meter.

Cochlear micromechanics

Acoustic signal processing occurs at the pinna, in the ear canal, and in the middle ear. Further mechanical processing occurs in the cochlea prior to neural encoding. Von Bekesy (1960) demonstrated that the peaks of the induced travelling waves in the inner ear are distributed tonotopically along the basilar membrane, causing its maximum excursion at a specific location. The travelling wave's velocity decreases from 30 m/s at the basal turn, to 1 m/s at the apex, and the whole journey takes from 2 to 5 ms, depending on whether the onset or the peak of the travelling wave is evaluated. High-frequency stimuli cause little motion of the basilar membrane beyond their point of maximum movement. However, low-frequency stimuli, causing maximum vibration more apically at a greater distance from the footplate of the stapes, also activate the basal portion of the basilar membrane. A click stimulus causes activation of the entire basilar membrane.

The process of frequency selectivity begins in the periphery, both at the basilar membrane and the hair cells, making the cochlea a basic spectral analyser. There is evidence to suggest that the stereocilia of different hair cells are mechanically tuned to the frequencies at which those cells respond, and that the height of the stereocilia is tonotopically organized (Tilney & Saunders 1983, Wright 1984, Saunders et al 1985). For example, in the alligator cochlea, a cell tuned to 1000 Hz has a stereociliary height of 30 μm, and a cell tuned to 400 Hz has a stereociliary height of 7 μm (Frishkopf & DeRosier 1983). However, the difference in the stereocilia has not been observed in man.

The single-unit primary neurone with its receptor field reveals a point of maximum sensitivity; and a frequency at which this phenomenon occurs is called a characteristic frequency (CF). The responsiveness to other fre-

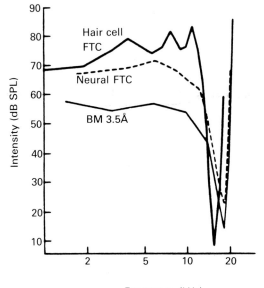

Fig. 2.4 Frequency tuning curves (FTC) in the guinea pig, showing mechanical basilar membrane displacement (BM 3.5×10^{-1} nm), inner hair cell voltage response (hair cell FTC), and auditory nerve fibre response (neural FTC). The tuning of all these elements is very similar. (Reproduced with permission from Pickles J O 1985.)

quencies is asymmetric and is greater towards the low frequencies. The plot of the threshold of a particular neurone responding to different frequencies is known as a frequency tuning curve (FTC), and the threshold is lowest at the CF (Fig. 2.4). The neurone responds best to stimuli at the CF, because its firing is governed by the inner hair cells at a particular place on the basilar membrane. This is seen in the finely tuned 'tip' of the FTC. The high-frequency portion of the 'tip' retains a steep slope but, on the low-frequency side, the slope changes to a lower value to form the 'tail' of the tuning curve. Figure 2.4 shows tuning curves for the amplitude displacement of the basilar membrane, and the neural tuning curve in a guinea pig which was obtained by Sellick et al (1982), and the data for hair cell FTC were obtained by Russell & Sellick (1978). Recent studies have indicated that mechanical tuning in the cochlea is close to neural tuning (Sellick et al 1982, Zwislocki 1985, Robles et al 1986).

Micromechanical transduction into electrical potentials starts in the cochlea. The hair cells and the cross-links among stereocilia are thought to be responsible for this phenomenon (Pickles et al 1984). There are transduction channels in the stereocilia for potassium current flow from the endolymph through the inner hair cells (Hudspeth 1985). These channels usually open when the stereocilia are bent in one direction, and close when they bend in the opposite direction. The vertical motion of the basilar membrane causes a relative horizontal shift between the tectorial membrane and the surface of the hair cells. It is thought that, at least, the tallest cilia of the outer cells are coupled to the bottom surface of the tectorial membrane, as shown in Figure 2.2. The cilia of the inner hair cells have no apparent contact with the tectorial membrane. Displacement of an area of the basilar membrane with hair cells causes a shearing motion of the stereocilia in contact with the tectorial membrane, and also produces a movement in relation to the endolymph (Tonndorf 1960). The latter movement produces a viscous drag on the unconnected cilia. This could suggest that outer hair cells, because of their cilia attachments, can be stimulated at lower sound intensities than can the inner hair cells with unattached cilia. The latter require considerably more sound intensity and endolymph movement. The shearing movement and bending of the stereocilia in the excitatory direction triggers the release of neurotransmitters in the synapses of the hair cells, and generates neural response (Dallos 1985). It is thought that the upward movement of the basilar membrane toward the scala vestibuli is excitatory, and that movement in the opposite direction is inhibitory.

It has been suggested that the inner ear also has the properties of an electromechanical transducer, and that oto-acoustic emissions from the cochlea can be recorded (Kemp 1978). It has been demonstrated that the oscillations of the membrane potential are coupled with the oscillations of the stereociliary bundle. This suggests that the inner hair cells are equipped to transduce not only mechanical energy into electrical, but also electrical oscillations of the potential of the cochlear partition into mechanical energy (Crawford & Fettiplace 1985).

Endocochlear potentials

An electrode introduced into the scala media and referred to an indifferent point enables the measurement of cochlear potentials. Endolymph with a high concentration of potassium and a low concentration of sodium registers an endolymphatic or endocochlear potential of +80 mV (von Békésy 1951). This positive extracellular resting potential is due not to a response to a stimulus, but to a metabolic activity produced by the stria vascularis. The hair cells also have an intracellular resting potential of −60 mV, otherwise known as a membrane potential, which exists in viable cells (Fig. 2.2). Using intracellular micro-electrode technique, Russell & Sellick (1978) succeeded in recording the intracellular potential in the mammalian cochlea. Davis (1965) suggested that the presence of endocochlear and intracellular potentials results in a voltage difference of about 140 mV across the surface of the hair cells, and this large potential is responsible for enhancing the excitability of the hair cells as a result of the presence of this high voltage gradient.

Receptor potentials

Mechanical deformation of the cilia alters the electrical resistance of the membrane. A sound stimulus creates changes of pressure and movement of the membrane, transforming current flow across the hair cells and cochlea fluids into alternating-current (AC) voltage. This stimulus-related potential, in a way, reproduces an instantaneous displacement pattern of the basilar membrane, and resembles the altered sound wave which has passed through the middle and inner ears. Wever & Bray (1930) recorded this potential in a cat, and it became known as the cochlear microphonic (CM). The CM is generated by the hair cells (Adrian 1931, Davis et al 1934).

Numerous further experimental and clinical studies have shown that destruction of the hair cells eliminates the CM (Dallos & Wang 1974). The main generators of the CM are the outer hair cells, the contribution from the inner hair cells being much smaller. As it is a receptor potential, the CM has practically no latency; in experiments on guinea pigs, it occurs with the delay of only 50 μs. When recorded with an extracochlear electrode, the CM represents the vectorial sum of the outputs of many hair cells with different magnitudes and, because of the distance to the electrode, with different phases (Fig. 2.5). When recorded from the promontory or the round window, the amplitude of the CM is several μV, and it grows linearly with increase of stimulus intensity until high levels of about 90 dB HTL, after which the transduction system of the cochlea becomes inefficient and exhibits non-linearities.

Another electrical phenomenon in response to sound stimulus is a direct-current (DC) potential. This can be recorded from the cochlea and was noted by Davis et al (1950). The DC change produced in the cochlea in response to a sound stimulus is known as the summating potential (SP). The SP has characteristics which are similar to the cochlear microphonic;

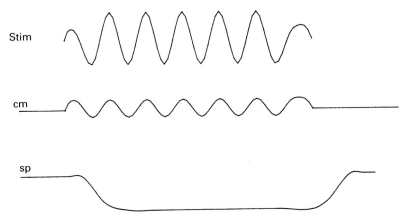

Stim

cm

sp

Fig. 2.5 Diagrammatic representation of the acoustic stimulus, cochlear microphonic, and summating potential.

it persists throughout the duration of the stimulus, its amplitude increases with increased stimulus intensity, and it does not fatigue at high repetition rates. The SP can be viewed as an electrical analogue of the mechano-electrical effects in the cochlea in response to acoustic stimulus.

The SP can be, at least partially, viewed as a non-linear distortion product of the hair cells' mechano-electrical transduction process, being produced when the hair cell membrane changes its resistance, and/or the basilar membrane moves more in one direction than another. This hypothesis was suggested by Davis et al (1952). Later Whitfield & Ross (1965), Eldredge (1974), and Dallos (1975) produced evidence for the conclusion that the SP results from the non-linearity of the CM generators. The amplitude and polarity of the SP depend upon the stimulus intensity and the frequency of the tone, as well as upon electrode location. The SP is a complex sum of several positive and negative components (Dallos 1973). Dallos et al (1972) and Dallos & Wang (1974) suggested that the positive SP(+) is produced by the outer hair cells and is more pronounced at relatively low sound-pressure levels. The negative SP(−) is generated from both the outer and inner hair cells at high-intensity levels.

Recording of the CM and SP from the round window or promontory in the normal human ear reveals that the CM is usually not symmetrical about the baseline and is superimposed on the negative SP.

The CM and SP could be important in further neural coding. Using intracellular micro-electrodes, Sellick & Russell (1978) have recorded the inner hair cells' CM and SP. They suggested that these potentials are associated with the activation of the fibres of the auditory nerve by a liberating neurotransmitter, which, in turn, stimulates neural connections to the hair cells.

Neurogenic potentials

Through synaptic transmission, the hair cells cause depolarization of the afferent dendrites of the cochlea nerve fibres. The first firing of the auditory nerve coincides with movement of the basilar membrane in the direction of the scala vestibuli, a movement which corresponds to the rarefaction phase of the stimulus (Kiang et al 1965). The spectral composition of the sound is transferred into tonotopically organized fibres, determining their neural pattern of activity. The auditory nerve fibres respond to tonal stimuli with two basic patterns of discharge; the first pattern is a sustained discharge with a peak rate at the onset of the tone, and the second pattern consists of activity locked in phase to the frequency of the tone. Sound intensity is coded in terms of the number of neurones activated and by the rate of firing within individual neurones.

The neurogenic potentials in response to auditory stimuli have a latent period and are of two types: spike action potentials (AP) and postsynaptic potentials (PSP).

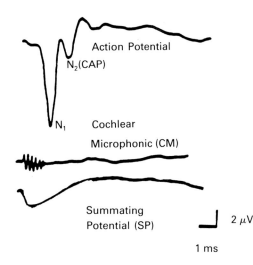

Fig. 2.6   The cochlear compound action potential (CAP) together with the CM and SP produced by a click stimulus.

The action potentials are generated at the cell body as spikes and transmitted along the axons to the cell's termination. The single-action potential has an all-or-none response to a stimulus and is associated with the onset or, sometimes, offset of a stimulus. A synchronized summation of neural discharges from the nerve cells and their axons produces a compound action potential (CAP) (see Fig. 2.6). The more neuronal units synchronized, the larger and better defined is the compound action potential (CAP). With increasing stimulus intensity, more neurones are activated. Even in their resting state, neurones still have a pattern of occasional random discharge. The compound action potential is dependent on synchrony of discharge and, therefore, on a fairly rapid onset of the acoustic stimulus. The absolute refractory period of the auditory neurones allows action potentials to be triggered at a rate of not more than about 400/s.

Following a synapse, dendrites can generate graded postsynaptic potentials. These potentials are less dependent on the synchrony of responses elicited by a fast onset acoustic stimulus. The dendritic potentials are topographically more localized in the nuclei, whilst the action potentials are active along the fibres. However, the latencies of stimulus-related potentials depend both on transduction along the fibres and on delay in the synaptic connections. Auditory evoked potentials are recorded from the scalp and are thought to be dominated by postsynaptic, rather than by spike action, potentials.

CLASSIFICATION OF THE AUDITORY EVOKED POTENTIALS

Auditory evoked potentials can reflect stimulus-related events in the cochlea, auditory nerve, brainstem, and cortex. By placing electrodes close to the generators, one can record in the near field of the potentials. For example, by using transtympanic electrocochleography and placing an electrode onto the promontory, one can record from the near field of the CAP.

Responses such as the CM can last throughout the stimulus duration, whilst the AP is transient, lasting only a few milliseconds. The responses may be divided into receptor, neurogenic, and myogenic potentials. The receptor potentials occur virtually instantaneously, whilst the neurogenic and myogenic potentials have latencies of up to 500 ms.

Neurogenic potentials can be divided into latency epochs (Picton et al 1974, Davis 1976, Jacobson & Hyde 1984), as shown in Figure 2.7 and Table 2.1. There are about 15 different auditory-evoked potentials.

The so-called 'early' potentials are generated in the cochlear nerve and the brainstem, and occur within the first 10 ms. They include the evoked potentials from the receptor organ and the cochlear nerve, which in normal subjects occur within the first few milliseconds. The so-called 'middle' latency responses occur within 8 to 50 ms and are generated in the thalamus and auditory cortex. The 'late' responses occur within 50 to 300 ms and are generated in the primary and secondary auditory cortex. There is a group of potentials called 'late' which is thought to originate in the primary and association areas of the cortex. These potentials occur at latencies greater than 300 ms.

For evoked potentials, there are several nomenclatures based on identification of the peaks and on their latencies. Davis (1976) has suggested the use of a polarity–latency convention. For example, the most prominent positive peak of the ABR, which occurs at 6 ms, is called P6 and corresponds

AVERAGED EVENT-RELATED POTENTIALS

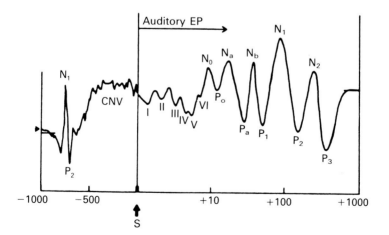

Fig. 2.7   Averaged neurogenic, post-signal, auditory-evoked potentials; early, middle, late (logarithmic scale), and pre-signal potential (CNV) associated with expectation (linear scale). (Reproduced with permission from Hillyard S A 1984.)

Table 2.1 Auditory evoked potentials

Name	Type	Latency	(ms)
Cochlear microphonic (CM)	Receptor		0
Summating potential (SP)	Receptor		0
Action potential (AP on ECochG: N1, N2, N3)	Neurogenic	Early	$\simeq 2$
Auditory brainstem response (ABR: I–VII)	Neurogenic	Early	<10
Slow negative (SN10)	Neurogenic	Early	$\simeq 10$
Frequency following response (FFR)	Neurogenic	Early	6
Middle latency response (MLR: No, Po, Na, Pa, Nb, Pb)	Neurogenic	Middle	8–50
Event-related potential (MLR–40 Hz)	Neurogenic	Middle	12–50
Postauricular muscle response (PAM)	Myogenic	Middle	$\simeq 16$
Slow vertex response (SVR: P1, N1, P2, N2)	Neurogenic	Middle	50–300
Sustained cortical potential (SCP)	Neurogenic	Middle	tone duration
Late positive component (P 300)	Neurogenic	Late	250–350
Contingent negative variation (CNV)	Neurogenic	Late	(−) 500

to wave V, according to the most commonly accepted nomenclature. The latencies vary according to stimulus intensity and temporal characteristics, as well as pathology. Accordingly, the sequential nomenclature designating the peaks, irrespective of the latency variability, is most commonly used for clinical purposes. The letters N and P indicate, respectively, negative or positive polarity. The designations N1 and N2 are used for negative peaks of the VIIIth nerve's action potential (AP). The roman numerals I to VII are used to label the major peaks of the 'fast' brainstem responses (ABR), as proposed by Jewett & Williston (1971). Less common is the use of arabic numerals, as proposed by Lev & Sohmer (1972). Middle-latency responses (MLR) are labelled No, Po, Na, Pa and Nb. The 'No' component of the MLR is identical to the slow negative wave in brainstem response which appears at about 10 ms and is known as SN10. Galambos et al (1981) has shown that the detectability of MLR is improved when a stimulus rate of 40/s is used. This response is known as '40 Hz MLR'. The SVR components are labelled P1, N1, P2 and N2. The small positive component, P1, is analogous to the Pb wave of the MLR.

The late-latency potentials occurring at about 300 ms, or later, and reflecting perceptual and cognitive activity are named P3 or P300. There is also a contingent negative variation (CNV), a pre-signal potential associated with expectancy.

The components starting from 75 ms and later, including N1, P2, N2 and P3, are highly sensitive to psychological variables, and some of them may depend on attention states or auditory information processing. They are called endogenous potentials. The earlier components do not depend upon psychological factors, and they are called exogenous potentials.

3. Basic principles of instrumentation and signal-processing

INTRODUCTION

The practising clinician does not need to know exactly how an evoked-potential (EP) system works, but he or she does need to know when it is not working. With familiar equipment such as an operating microscope, the same principle holds, but in this case it is easy to tell when the equipment is not working. If the image cannot be clearly focused, there is obviously a problem: if, however, the microscope should give a perfectly clear image but one showing abnormal anatomy when the patient being examined is normal, then such a fault could not easily be detected. It is a principle of basic optics that such a problem cannot occur with a microscope, but exactly that problem can happen with an evoked-potential system.

When being tested with auditory-evoked potentials, the patient is connected to the system, stimulated with sound, and produces a response. Diagnostic inferences are then made, based upon that response. If the equipment is not set up correctly, it is possible that the response will be determined more by the physics of sampling and filtering than by the physiology of the patient. Once the response has been obtained, there may be no way of knowing whether equipment errors have been responsible for the final waveform. The clinician is left with a response which will be interpreted in the light of other clinical data in order to make a diagnosis. It is, therefore, important to know the basic principles of an EP system, to be aware of the important factors in setting up the equipment so that valid diagnoses can be made, and to know how such systems can be checked and calibrated.

The basic task of the recording system is to extract small amplitude EPs from other electrical signals recorded from the same site. As the EP is the signal of interest, all other electrical waveforms may be regarded as interference and contamination of the record. In some instances, an EP of 1 μV will be contained within a recording which has 50 μV of electrical activity as a result of physiologic signals or electrode-contact potentials, and it is important to maximize the signal-to-noise ratio (S/N) of the EP. All the elements in an EP recording system play a part in improving the signal-to-noise ratio.

BASIC RECORDING TECHNIQUES

Electrodes

In this section, only surface electrodes will be considered. Although needle and other electrodes are used for recording some EPs, these will be detailed when the appropriate response is considered.

It is at the surface of the scalp that the S/N ratio is worst for a surface-recorded EP. Therefore, some care should be taken in the choice of electrodes, in their placement, and in the technique used for attaching them to the scalp. Poor electrode technique can worsen the S/N ratio still further, and, clearly, such an effect must be minimized.

An electrode in contact with the skin generates a contact potential which substantially adds to the noise from which the EP must be extracted. The electrical impedance of the electrode/skin junction not only plays a part in determining the value of the contact potential, but also determines the noise generated by the electrode and the magnitude of induced electromagnetic artefacts. Clearly, the contact impedance of the electrode must be kept low in order to minimize these effects.

Prior to attaching the electrode, one should prepare the skin surface by vigorous rubbing with spirit or acetone. This removes grease and layers of dead skin, and reduces the electrode/skin contact impedance.

The electrode material is the major factor determining the contact potential. Silver has a low contact potential, and further improvements can be made by using a fluid-column electrode in which the electrode itself does not touch the skin, the connection being made by a saline solution or electrode jelly. The noise generated by the electrode is predominantly low-frequency, and this noise may be reduced by using a reversible electrode, such as silver coated with silver chloride.

Again at low frequencies, the electrode may cause distortion because of the capacitance that its contact with the skin produces. The distortion caused by this electrode capacitance is very small for silver/silver chloride electrodes.

The electrode contact with the skin should be tested with an alternating-current impedance meter. This measure is one that varies with the frequency at which it is taken, and so a 'good contact' can be represented by an impedance of 2000 Ω measured at 1000 Hz, or by an impedance of 4000 Ω measured at 20 Hz. Both of these figures can represent the same degree of contact between the electrode and the skin. It is important, therefore, to be aware of the frequency at which the impedance meter tests the electrodes. Many commercial systems have built-in impedance meters, and, in general, these use a frequency of around 50 Hz. For reasons that will be given in the next section, it is important that the impedances of each electrode pair should be as similar as possible. It is better to achieve balanced impedances than to have only one electrode with a very low impedance. Direct-current test meters should never be used to measure electrode contact. This can polarize the electrodes, adding to the noise they produce, and, more significantly, currents in excess of the present safety limits could be passed through the patient.

It is common practice to place the recording electrodes in the standard position defined by the international 10–20 system for electroencephalography (Jasper 1958). Currently, there is no generally accepted form for presenting the waveform recorded from an electrode pair. For many of the auditory-evoked potentials, both electrodes are 'active' and will register some of the response. The choice of which electrode represents the positive input to the amplifier is therefore an arbitrary one, and examples of both the possible waveform polarities may be found in the literature. It should be recognized that changes in electrode position can result in changes in waveform morphology, latency, and amplitude.

Differential amplification

As its name implies, a differential amplifier is one whose output is equal to the difference between two input voltages. Thus, for two input voltages A and B, the output of the amplifier is G(A–B) where G is the gain of the amplifier. Such an amplifier can improve the S/N ratio in the following way. The unwanted background noise, predominantly the EEG, is very nearly the same signal at many places on the scalp. If a pair of electrodes are positioned such that much of the noise is the same at both electrodes but the EP presents predominantly to only one of the positions, then when the signals from the pair of electrodes are fed into a differential amplifier, the noise that is common to the two electrodes will be cancelled, whilst the EP will be largely unchanged. Assuming, for the sake of simplicity, that the EP presents only to electrode A with a voltage Ea, then the two signals at A and B are, respectively, (A)=Ea+Nc+Na and (B)=Nc+Nb, where Na and Nb are the lesser amounts of noise that differ between position A and position B, and Nc is the greater amount of noise that is common to the two electrodes. The output of the differential amplifier is Ea with the two noise components Na and Nb, and so the S/N ratio has been improved by the elimination of the common noise Nc. The degree to which a differential amplifier can cancel common noise is called its common-mode rejection ratio (CMRR). This should be of the order of 100 dB, meaning that voltages which are identical at the input will be attenuated by 100 dB at the output.

If the impedance of one electrode is very much less than that of the other, the differential amplifier is no longer balanced and its CMRR will be decreased. Thus, for good noise reduction, it is important to keep the contact impedances of the electrodes as similar as possible.

The electrode/skin junction provides a capacitive connection between the signal generated on the scalp and that passed to the differential amplifier. This capacitance, combined with the input impedance of the differential amplifier, can create a filter which will distort the recorded waveform. To ensure that any such distortion occurs only at a frequency that is outside the frequency range of the response, the input impedance of the amplifier should be very high; generally, of the order of 10 MΩ.

Wires that are terminated in a high impedance are prone to pick up electromagnetic signals from external sources. Thus, the electrode leads should be kept as short as possible, and the differential amplifier placed close to the patient. The main amplifier may then be placed at some distance from the patient, provided that the output impedance of the differential amplifier is low enough that the wires leading from the differential amplifier to the main amplifier do not pick up significant amounts of interference.

Thus, the pre-amplifier of an EP system must be a differential amplifier to reduce common noise, have a high input impedance to minimize distortion, have a low output impedance so that the leads to the main amplifier do not pick up electromagnetic interference, and be placed close to the patient so that the electrode leads can be short. There is no requirement for a large gain at this stage, and the gain of the pre-amplifier is generally less than 10. Most of the actual amplification is carried out in the main amplifier.

Band-pass filtering

A filter, as its name implies, is a device which permits some frequencies to pass through unattenuated while filtering out others. A band-pass filter is one that will allow through frequencies lying within a certain range. The high and low cut-off frequencies of the band are described by the frequency at which the attenuation of the filter has reached 3 dB. Figure 3.1 shows a typical band-pass filter characteristic. The lower cut-off frequency is marked as f1, and the higher as f2. For frequencies lower than f1 or higher than f2, an increasing amount of attenuation is created by the filter. The steepness of the filter characteristic in these regions is known as the filter slope and is expressed in dB/octave.

The spectrum of a signal describes the amplitude of the different frequency components contained within that signal. A pure sine wave has only one component at the frequency of the wave. However, signals such as evoked responses have many components of different amplitudes and frequencies.

In general, the spectrum of the background noise is wider than that of the response. This is illustrated in Figure 3.2(A), in which the signal-to-noise ratio is represented by the ratio of the area delineated by the vertical lines to that delineated by the horizontal lines. Thus, there are frequency regions which contain only noise and no significant response-components. If the signal is passed through a band-pass filter whose characteristics are set such that the spectrum of the response is not modified, then those frequency regions containing only noise can be eliminated and the S/N ratio improved. Figure 3.2(B) shows a filter characteristic, and the resultant spectra which

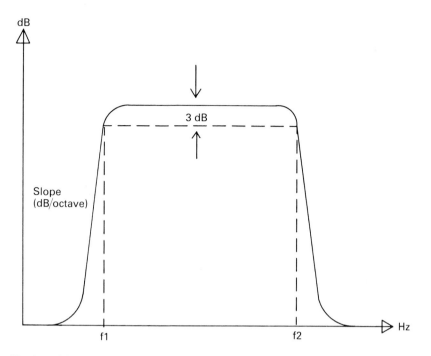

Fig. 3.1 A band-pass filter transfer function. Gain, in dB, is shown on the vertical axis and frequency on the horizontal axis. The '3-dB-down' cut-off points are shown for the lower frequency (f1) and the higher frequency (f2). The slope of the skirts of the filter is measured in dB/octave.

appear at the output of the filter are shown in Figure 3.2(C). The ratio of the areas of the response spectrum to the noise spectrum has now been significantly increased.

As the filter bandwidth is narrowed, the S/N ratio for the response improves. However, at some frequency, the band limits begin to filter out the response spectrum, eliminate components of the response, and hence distort the waveform and reduce response amplitude. Figure 3.3 shows the effects of different recording bandwidths on the post-auricular muscle (PAM) response, and it can be seen that the response is markedly altered. Clearly, the band limits have to be chosen with considerable care.

Physicists are often concerned with setting filter limits to preserve waveform fidelity. However, clinically, one does not have to be unduly concerned with this idea. In clinical practice, maximum waveform fidelity is an arbitrary concept involving considerations of what is the 'true' response and whether the eliminated frequency components are a clinically significant part of the response. If the response is to be used for threshold estimation, then maximum response detectability is required, and waveform distortion is not important. Thus, for this application, filter limits should be chosen to maximize response detectability rather than for any other reason. Only

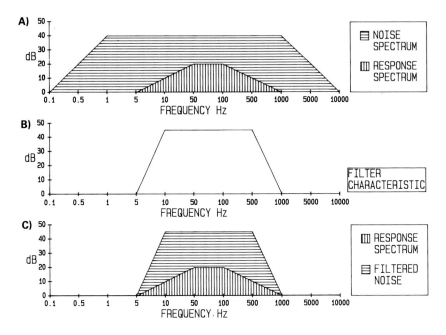

Fig. 3.2 Improvement of signal-to-ratio by band-pass filtering. (**A**) shows the general case in which the spectrum of the noise covers a greater frequency range than does the spectrum of the response. The signal-to-noise ratio is represented by the area delineated by the vertical lines divided by that delineated by the horizontal lines. After being passed through a band-pass filter with the characteristics shown in (**B**), the resultant spectra are shown in (**C**). The signal-to-noise ratio is now clearly improved.

if there is diagnostic information to be obtained from the waveform of the response should the filter limits be set such that the waveform is not distorted.

The filter will also introduce a propagation delay which increases as the bandwidth becomes narrower. If no allowance is made for this delay, then the response latencies may be in error by the amount of the propagation delay. This may be easily checked by using a click stimulus and connecting the electrical signal at the headphones via an attenuator to the input pre-amplifiers. The latency of the stimulus should, of course, be 0 and any discrepancy from this value is most probably an indication that the equipment has not allowed for filter-propagation delays. Such discrepancies have been seen in commercially produced equipment.

Limiting and rejection

Limiting, or peak clipping, involves restricting the input signal to pre-set voltage limits. If these limits are set such that the signal is unaltered for most of the time that the patient is generating low levels of physiologic noise, then occasional, high-amplitude signals will cause the limiter to

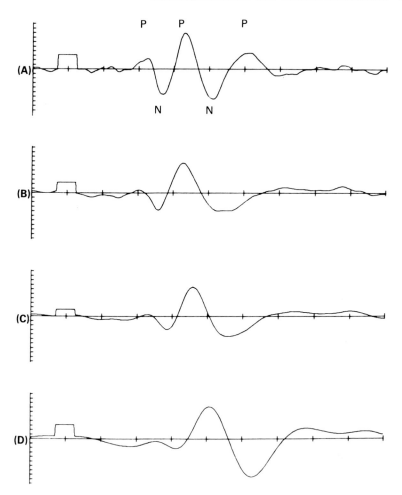

Fig. 3.3   Effects of filter bandwidth on the postauricular muscle response. The change in waveforms with various high-frequency limits is shown. The limits are (**A**) 4 kHz, (**B**) 500 Hz, (**C**) 200 Hz, and (**D**) 100 Hz (x axis = 5 ms/div.; y axis = 0.5 μV/div.).

operate. This ensures that the amplitude of the input signal, during these particularly noisy periods, is not as great as it could have been. Protecting the recorded signal from large-amplitude noise values will, clearly, improve the S/N ratio. A more sophisticated approach is to reject any signal epochs in which the EEG has exceeded the pre-set values. This means that the response will be taken from only the low-noise periods in the recording.

TIME-DOMAIN AVERAGING

Time-domain averaging is the single, most powerful technique for improving the S/N ratio of the response.

Theory of operation

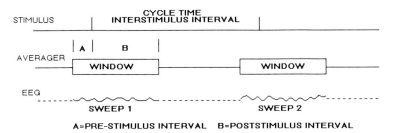

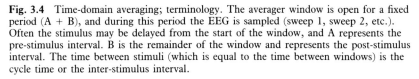

Fig. 3.4   Time-domain averaging; terminology. The averager window is open for a fixed period (A + B), and during this period the EEG is sampled (sweep 1, sweep 2, etc.). Often the stimulus may be delayed from the start of the window, and A represents the pre-stimulus interval. B is the remainder of the window and represents the post-stimulus interval. The time between stimuli (which is equal to the time between windows) is the cycle time or the inter-stimulus interval.

Figure 3.4 illustrates the terminology used in describing the operation of an averager. A section of the amplified signal from the electrodes is sampled, using an analogue-to-digital converter (ADC). This measures the voltage of the input signal at an instant in time, and converts this voltage into a numerical value which is stored in a location in the averager memory. Many samples are taken at short time intervals until the required section of input signal has been sampled and stored. In this way, a digital representation of a section of the input signal is placed in the averager memory. This section is called a sweep, and the duration of the section is known as the window used by the averager. The timing relationship between stimulus and recording system is critical. The stimulus may be presented at the start of the window or, as shown here, at a fixed time after the start of the window. This allows a pre-stimulus interval with which any response occurring in the post-stimulus interval of the window can be compared. Some time after the window has finished, the cycle is repeated and the time between windows is known as the cycle time, which is, of course, equal to the inter-stimulus interval. At the end of the second sweep, the values of this sweep are added to those obtained from the first sweep, and, as more sweeps are acquired, their sum is gradually accumulated.

Figure 3.5 illustrates how this accumulation improves the S/N ratio. A single sweep, stored in memory, may be considered as comprising two parts, shown in the top half of Figure 3.5. The first part is the response, or signal, and the second is noise. In this figure, an artificial signal has been added to real EEG noise to illustrate the averaging process. For a fixed set of stimulus parameters, it is assumed that the response is constant and so the timing relationship among the window, the stimulus, and the response will remain fixed. Thus, when values from successive sweeps are added to the values obtained from the first sweep, the response will always occur at the same point in the sweep (time-locked), and its amplitude will increase

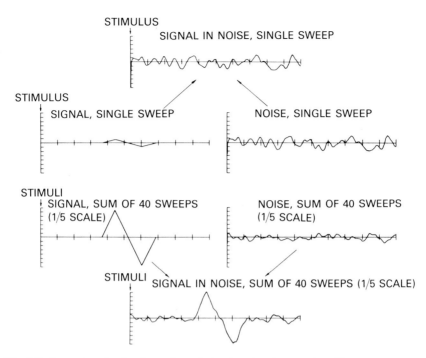

Fig. 3.5 Improving the signal-to noise ratio by time-domain averaging. The top trace represents what is recorded in a single sweep, that is, the response buried in noise. Below, the response and noise have been separated to illustrate the averaging process. The next pair of traces shows, again separately, the response or signal and the noise after 40 sweeps have been summed. The signal will grow linearly to 40 times its original magnitude, whereas the noise will be much less than 40 times its original magnitude. The combination of these two traces produces the bottom waveform, which is what would be recorded on an averager after 40 sweeps.

linearly with the number of sweeps. The noise processes are, of course, not time-locked to the stimulus, and, at a point in the window, the noise can take any value, positive or negative, for different sweeps. Clearly, the noise values are not going to add linearly in the same way as the response because sometimes they will tend to cancel and sometimes they will add. More correctly, it can be shown that the noise will add according to a root–mean–square (rms) rule.

The enhancement of the S/N ratio by this factor of the square root of the number of sweeps will occur only if the assumptions of an invariant response and a normally distributed random noise are met. To the relief of the neurologist and others who use EEG patterns diagnostically, the EEG is not strictly a normally distributed random noise. However, for EP work, the EEG approximates adequately to this assumption, which means that after 100 sweeps the S/N ratio has improved by a factor of 10, and after 2500 sweeps, by a factor of 50.

Commercial averagers are now computer-based systems and automatically provide facilities such as buffered averaging, which allows high-noise level sweeps to be rejected. For this, a sweep is acquired and temporarily stored in a reserved section of memory. The values may then be examined automatically, and, if the limits are exceeded, this sweep will not be added to the main average. Only if the limits are not exceeded is the sweep added to the accumulating sum. Generally, there is a display of the number of rejected sweeps and that of accepted sweeps so that the operator can adjust the limits if necessary.

Sampling

The ADC converts the analogue voltage of the input signal into a binary number. The minimum step size depends upon the number of digits allowed in this binary number; this is illustrated in Figure 3.6 for a three-digit binary number with $8(2^3)$ steps. This quantization, or digital conversion, of the signal introduces sampling errors, as the fixed levels available from the ADC do not correspond exactly to the actual voltage level of the signal. In practice, ADCs use 8- to 12-digit numbers, which adequately represent the signals being considered here.

A more important consideration is the sampling rate. If a sweep has been sampled 200 times by the ADC for a window of 20 ms, then the sample rate is 10 000 samples/s. It is important to know if this sample rate is one that is adequate and will avoid errors.

The correct sample rate is related to the highest frequency present in the input signal, and it is a common fallacy to relate the sample rate to the highest frequency of interest to the operator. For a simple signal, such as

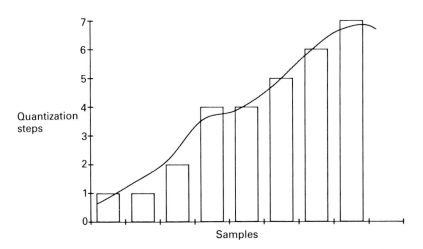

Fig. 3.6 Illustration of analogue-to-digital conversion. The smooth line represents the voltage of the analogue waveform and the discrete digital sample values are shown for a three-bit ADC which has eight quantization steps.

a sine wave, it can be shown that if it is sampled at a rate which is greater than two samples per period of the sine wave, then the samples will uniquely define the signal, and there will be no error. Any signal, such as an EEG, may be considered to comprise a set of sine waves of different amplitudes and frequencies. Therefore, if the EEG is sampled at a rate which is greater than two samples per period for the highest frequency component present, then all lower-frequency elements will have been more than adequately sampled, and this will ensure that the EEG signal is correctly digitized by the averager.

If the sample rate is not high enough, the signal will not be accurately recorded, and distortion of the waveform and hence of the final average can occur. Such errors are known as aliasing errors, and there is no way of determining from the averaged waveform that such errors have occurred. It is, therefore, important to prevent their occurrence, and this is done by the high-frequency limit set on the band-pass filter. This must limit the high-frequency end of the signal spectrum so that the conditions mentioned above are met. It is unnecessary to detail the mathematical equation governing this relationship, but the clinician should ensure that the technical staff involved are aware of these factors.

STIMULUS GENERATION

Stimuli

The choice of stimulus depends upon the EP to be recorded and the desired clinical objective. If pure-tone thresholds (hearing threshold level [HTL]) are to be estimated, then, clearly, tone bursts, similar to those used in subjective audiometry, appear to be a logical choice for the stimulus, as they have a narrow spectrum and are, hence, frequency specific. However, it should be noted that frequency-specific stimuli do not always produce frequency-specific EP responses. Furthermore, the use of a long-duration stimulus when a short-latency response is being recorded can give a false impression. Clearly, all of the stimulus that occurs after the response has been generated can have no further influence on that response. Therefore, tone bursts or tone pips of a duration which is comparable to the latency of the response being measured are used. Figure 3.7 illustrates the spectra associated with tone bursts, tone pips, and clicks.

The shorter the duration of a tone burst, the wider will be the spread of frequencies contained within its spectrum. Furthermore, onset transients must be reduced by having a smooth rise-and-fall envelope to shape the tone burst. However, the rise time of the stimulus must be short enough to provide sufficient neural synchrony for adequate response generation, particularly for the early responses.

For these short-latency responses, the stimulus that gives the best neural synchrony and hence the largest response amplitude is a click. This is

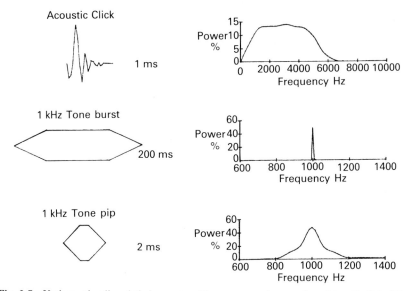

Fig. 3.7 Various stimuli and their spectra. The top trace shows a 'broad-band' click. The middle trace is a 1 kHz tone burst, as used in conventional audiometry. The bottom trace shows a short-duration tone pip.

commonly produced by passing a rectangular voltage pulse of 100 μs duration to the earphone. The polarity of the click is often referred to by the acoustic waveform that it produces. A pulse that initially moves the earphone diaphragm towards the eardrum is known as a condensation click, and the opposite polarity, which moves the diaphragm away from the eardrum, is known as a rarefaction click. It should be noted that applying a voltage pulse of the same polarity and in the same way to the terminals of different earphones does not guarantee on acoustic output of the same polarity. The internal wiring of earphones can differ among units produced by the same manufacturer. The polarity of the acoustic output should be checked, and several investigators have described ways of doing this (Staewen et al 1980, Salt & Thornton 1983).

EPs may also be produced by bone-conducted stimuli. A conventional bone-conductor may be used in place of the earphones, but there are problems in recording the early responses. Firstly, the click waveform is severely degraded by the bone-conductor and loses much of its high-frequency content. Secondly, the bone-conductor produces a large electromagnetic artefact which contaminates much of the set of early response peaks. Special techniques can be applied to overcome this problem partially, but, in general clinical practice, bone-conducted stimuli are used only to elicit the middle- and long-latency responses.

Stimulus calibration

Stimuli that are the same as those used in normal audiometric practice can be calibrated by standard procedures; otherwise, a 'biological' calibration can be carried out, using a group of normally hearing subjects. Most of the stimuli used in EP work require this 'biological' calibration. At least 10 normally hearing subjects should be used, and the stimuli should be delivered at the same rate as in routine testing.

Once the norms have been determined for a particular EP system, stimulus levels may be set appropriately. There are no international standards for the physical calibration of short-duration stimuli, and it has become common practice to describe the stimulus level with reference to the threshold for normally hearing subjects. This is expressed as dBnHL and provides a satisfactory solution in the clinic.

This biological calibration is too lengthy a procedure to repeat at regular intervals in order to check that the equipment remains within calibration, and so some physical measure of sound pressure level (SPL) is also needed. The most commonly accepted one is decibel peak equivalent sound pressure level (dBpeSPL), and this may be measured in the following way. The earphone is placed on an artificial ear (e.g. Bruel & Kjaer type 4152), the output of the artificial ear is fed into a sound level meter (SLM) (e.g. Bruel & Kjaer type 2203), and the electrical output of the SLM is connected to an oscilloscope. Clicks at a nominal level of about 70 dB SPL are fed into the earphone, but the reading, if any, on the SLM should be ignored at this stage. The oscilloscope should be adjusted to display the click and the peak-to-peak amplitude measured. A pure tone, generally at 3 kHz, is then fed into the earphone, and its amplitude adjusted to give the same peak-to-peak amplitude reading on the oscilloscope. The SLM is then read to obtain the peak-equivalent sound-pressure level of the click. Again using the oscilloscope, one can record the time intervals between the start of the click and the two successive zero crossings. These data should provide an adequate check that the equipment remains within its initial calibration values and gives the necessary measurements for any adjustments that are needed.

OVERALL SYSTEM

Figure 3.8 shows an overall block diagram of a basic, two-channel EP system. The signal from the electrodes is amplified by the pre-amplifier and then passed to the main amplifier, which may also contain the band-pass filters. The amplified signal is then passed to the limiter and on to the averager. The stimulus generator provides the test signals, which are passed, via attenuators, to the output transducers, such as loudspeakers, earphones, or bone conductors. White noise should also be provided for masking, and there must be a timing link between the stimulus generator and

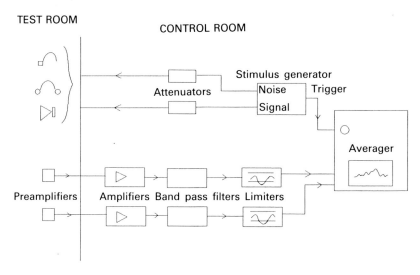

Fig. 3.8 Block diagram of a basic auditory-evoked response system.

the averager to ensure correct triggering. Many commercial systems provide a complete package, and, with modern computer technology, the limiting and rejection is done on the digitized waveform within the computer.

The test environment will depend upon the type of EP to be measured, whether anaesthetic facilities are required, and the particular needs of the clinic. With modern equipment, there is usually no need for electromagnetically screened rooms, although, clearly, soundproofing is required if threshold measurements are to be taken.

Other systems and techniques have been developed, but have not yet achieved routine application in clinical practice. Using a superconducting quantum interference device (SQUID), one can record the magnetic fields associated with evoked potentials. Such a recording system offers potential benefits to fundamental research, but, so far, has shown no significant advantage that would outweigh the cost, technical difficulties, and clinical awkwardness of using supercooled detection equipment.

CLINICAL AND TECHNICAL CONSIDERATIONS

Manipulation of the averaged response

Several basic techniques may be used to manipulate the averaged response. Perhaps the most common of these is the facility to add and subtract averaged responses that have been recalled from a backing store or are in different areas of the averager's memory. Such a facility provides the means to carry out derived-response techniques, as well as, for example, the separation of cochlear microphonic, action potential, and summating potential responses in a transtympanic electrocochleographic recording (Eggermont &

Odenthal 1974). An example is shown in Figure 3.9, in which waveform A is an abnormal EP combined with the summating potential recorded at a rate of 5 stimuli per second. The abnormality may be due to the action potential (AP) or to the summating potential (SP). A second recording was then made (trace B) at 100 stimuli per second, which ensured that the AP component had been maximally adapted and would make virtually no contribution to the recorded waveform. Thus, waveform B represents the SP component alone. The subtraction of B from A, shown in waveform C, gives a normal AP and demonstrates that the abnormality is due to an abnormal SP.

Techniques such as smoothing, demeaning, and detrending are also clinically useful. Smoothing the trace reduces small irregularities on the waveform and often makes peak detection easier. Whilst helping pattern recognition, it does modify, to some degree, the waveform, and so measurements should be taken from waveforms that have been smoothed only a little or not at all. Demeaning sets the mean value of the wave to zero and removes the effects of any DC shifts. In a similar way, detrending removes from the waveform the effects of linear trends in the record, and, therefore,

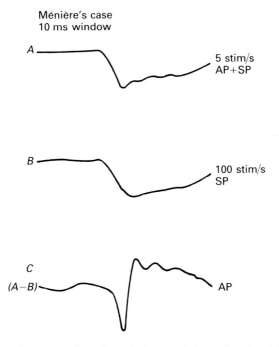

Fig. 3.9   The use of memory subtraction techniques. (**A**) shows the AP and SP trace recorded at 5 stimuli/s. (**B**) shows a response that is predominantly SP, the AP having been adapted by using a stimulus rate of 100 stimuli/s. (**C**) is the AP obtained by subtracting **B** from **A**. This is quite characteristic for a Ménière's disease case in which the abnormality in the AP/SP complex is due to the SP.

gives a better definition of the waveform; but, particularly with some EPs, this technique should be used with care.

Masking techniques

Contralateral masking according to the normal audiometric rules may be used to ensure monaural stimulation (Reid & Thornton 1983). Broad-band or white noise-masking should be used for a click stimulus.

Filtered masking noise, mixed with the stimulus and presented to the test ear, can be used to improve the frequency specificity of both clicks and short-duration tones. Figure 3.10 illustrates the principles involved in the two methods. To eliminate the high-frequency components in a click or tone burst, one can use masking as shown in Figure 3.10(A). This technique has been used by Kileny (1981) and Laukli (1983).

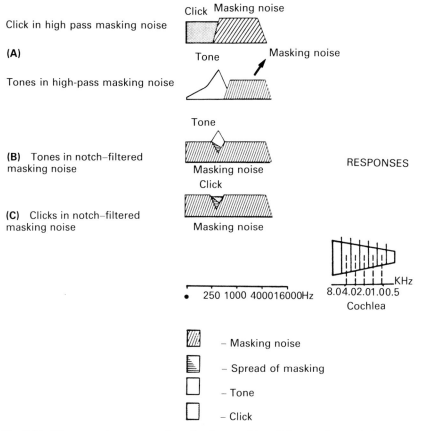

Fig. 3.10 Diagrammatic representation of various masking click strategies to obtain more frequency-specific responses. (**A**) Clicks and tones. (**B**) presented with high-pass masking noise. (**C**) A tone in notch-filtered masking noise. (**D**) A click presented in notch-filtered masking noise.

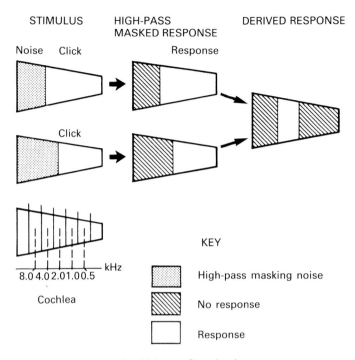

Fig. 3.11 Derived-responses using high-pass filtered noise.

The notch noise-masking technique, illustrated in Figure 3.10(B) for tones and in Figure 3.10(C) for a click, has been used by Eggermont & Odenthal (1974) and by Picton et al (1979). Here the masking noise is broad-band, except for a small notch in which the stimulus can produce a response with a limited frequency range. The responses to notch-masked tones are usually more frequency-specific and larger than are the responses obtained using a click stimulus, according to Stapells et al (1985). The technique has been validated on selected patients and does improve the frequency selectivity, but recent data, obtained using click stimuli in notch noise, have shown large errors in estimating hearing thresholds at specific frequencies, indicating that this approach has some limitations (Pratt et al 1984).

The derived-response technique was introduced by Tease et al (1962) and uses a broad-band click stimulus with a series of high-pass masking noises. The principle is illustrated in Figure 3.11, and each derived-response is obtained as follows. With the high-pass masker set to a cut-off frequency of f2 Hz, the click stimulus produces a response from the 0 to f2 Hz frequency region of the auditory system. This response is recorded and stored. The high-pass masker is then set to a lower cut-off frequency (f1 Hz). The click now elicits a response from the 0 to f1 Hz region of the auditory system. Subtracting the second response waveform from the first response waveform gives the 'narrow-band', or derived-response, from the region f1–f2 Hz.

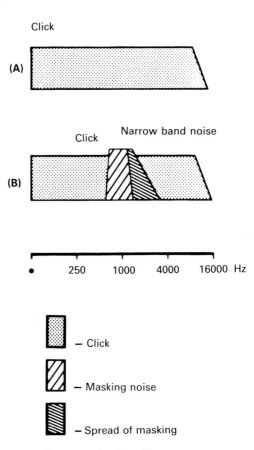

Fig. 3.12   Derived-response using narrow-band masking

Parker & Thornton (1978c) validated the use of this technique with ABR and checked that the derived band did correspond to the high-pass filtered setting (Parker & Thornton 1978b). The technique has also been applied in electrocochleography (Elberling 1974) and in ABR by Don & Eggermont (1978).

A more complicated method of derived-response using narrow-band masking may be obtained by using a specific masking tone or a narrow-band noise (Fig. 3.12). First, by simultaneous presentation of click and narrow-band masking noise, the generation of the response contribution from the masked place is suppressed (B). Next, response (A) is recorded to click only. By subtracting response A from response B, a derived-response will be obtained, representing the place of masked area of the cochlea (Stapells et al 1984).

Frequency-domain aspects

In averaging a waveform, the averager will also, in a very particular way, filter the signal. This aspect of averaging can be used to eliminate fixed-frequency contaminating waveforms, such as mains hum, and can even be used to eliminate electrophysiological signals which remain fairly constant, such as alpha rhythm. As explained earlier, the averager improves the S/N ratio for signals that are time-locked to the window. If a fixed-cycle time is used, then signals that are time-locked to the cycle time will also have their S/N ratio improved. Because any signal may be regarded as being made up of sine waves of different frequencies and amplitudes, there can be components which are time-locked to the cycle time of the averager. The frequency components that have a period of a duration that fits once or several times exactly into the cycle time are added linearly by the averager, and the S/N ratio for these components improved in the same way as the response. In contrast, frequency components that have one-half a period or an odd number of half-periods that fit exactly into the cycle time will be present in one phase for odd-numbered sweeps and in the opposite phase for even-numbered sweeps, and will thus cancel out in the average. This fact does not invalidate averaging; it is merely a frequency-domain representation of the events for which the time-domain aspects were detailed earlier (p. 28). However, this aspect may be put to good use in the clinic. If mains hum interferes with the recording, it may be eliminated. In the UK, the mains frequency is 50 Hz, and so the period is 20 ms. If the averager cycle time is set so that it is an odd multiple of 10 ms (the half-period), then any mains hum picked up in the recording will be cancelled by the averager. In a similar manner, when one is recording the slow vertex response, if the patient's alpha rhythm is a problem, this can be extracted through a filter and used to trigger the averager on a positive peak for odd-numbered sweeps and on a negative peak for even-numbered sweeps such that the alpha rhythm will be cancelled in the average.

Clinical use of auditory evoked potentials

4. Electrocochleography (ECochG)

INTRODUCTION

Electrocochleography (ECochG), a recording of electrical activity generated in the cochlea and the auditory nerve, can provide useful information about inner-ear function. The main clinical application of ECochG is in the estimation of hearing threshold, especially in children who are difficult to test with behavioural audiometry. These include very young children, those who are actively non-cooperative, and the mentally and physically handicapped. Abnormal ECochG patterns may also reflect pathological changes in the cochlea or auditory nerve.

GENERATORS OF COCHLEAR AND VIIITH NERVE POTENTIALS

Auditory-evoked potentials from the receptor organ (CM and SP) and the action potential (AP) of the VIIIth nerve can be recorded using the near-field recording method of electrocochleography (Fig. 4.1). The CM and SP

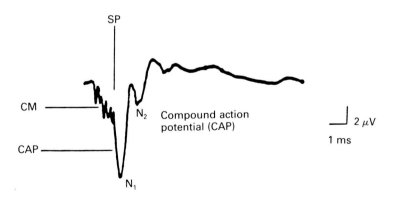

Fig. 4.1 Cochlear and VIIIth nerve potentials in response to a monophasic click. The CM appears on the leading edge of the SP response.

occur virtually without delay, and the AP occurs within the first few milliseconds after the stimulus onset for high-level click stimuli.

Both the alternating-current response (CM) and the direct-current response (SP) are sustained potentials persisting throughout the stimulus duration, and reflect mechano-electrical events in the cochlea. Like the SP, the CM is seen most clearly in response to pure tones. The CM is usually not symmetric about the baseline and is superimposed on the negative SP.

The main contribution to the gross CM and SP recorded transtympanically comes predominantly from the output of the outer hair cells at the basal end. This is partly due to the fact that the number of outer hair cells is about three times the number of inner hair cells.

The AP is best elicited in response to abrupt, transient sounds such as a broad-band click, which activates the neural fibres in synchrony (Fig. 4.1). Within a few milliseconds, the activity in the fibres returns to their normal, random, very low rate of discharge, and the AP is not observed. It can be shown (Kiang, Moxon & Kahn 1976) that the AP is the convolution integral of the single-fibre impulses. Thus, the surface-recorded or compound AP reflects both the number of fibres activated and the degree of synchrony among them. The highest speed of the travelling wave propagation is in the basal turn, and, therefore, the synchronization of the AP is greatest at the high-frequency region of the cochlea. Travelling wave propagation towards the apical part of the cochlea and progressive time delay creates out-of-phase responses of individual fibres with less synchrony. Therefore, the contributions from more apical regions are more difficult to record.

In man, the compound AP shows two or three negative peaks (N1, N2, and sometimes N3) which are thought to be recorded from the nerve up to the level of the medial part of the internal auditory meatus. However, in small laboratory mammals, in which the VIIIth nerve is much shorter, the N1 potential recorded from the promontory represents a synchronized response from the auditory nerve, and the N2 peak represents response from the neurones of the cochlear nucleus (Ruben et al 1982, Moller 1983).

METHODS

Testing environment

Avoidance of both electrical interference and excessive muscular activity is essential in order to obtain good signal-to-noise ratios, and to record the responses close to the hearing threshold. Testing in a quiet environment is desirable, and an anechoic chamber is the ideal acoustic environment for free-field testing.

The patient is tested while lying quietly on a couch. For adult patients who can be trusted to keep their heads still and not turn onto the needle electrode, a local anaesthetic can be used. But in children, general anaesthesia and, hence, an operating theatre are needed.

Electrode placement

Cochlear microphonics from the round window of man were first recorded during surgery by Fromm et al (1935) and Gersuni et al (1937). Later, Ruben et al (1959, 1961, 1967) and Ronis (1966) recorded CM and AP by using a surgical approach to the round window.

At present, two main techniques are used to record ECochG in clinical practice. One technique is the transtympanic method, in which a needle electrode is placed on the promontory, and the other technique is to use an extratympanic electrode placed in the external auditory meatus (Fig. 4.2).

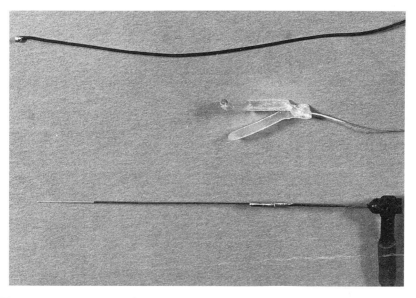

Fig. 4.2   Transtympanic needle electrode (botom), an extratympanic electrode (middle), and silver ball electrode (top) which may be used to record either from the round window or the annulus.

As this is a near-field recording technique, the position of the reference electrode is not critical. Usually a surface silver/silver chloride electrode is placed on the ipsilateral ear lobe or the mastoid. For extratympanic electrocochleography, some investigators use the contralateral ear lobe or mastoid as a reference position. The ground electrode is usually placed on the forehead.

The transtympanic method was attempted by Lempert (1950) and successfully developed and popularized by Portmann (1968). The sterile needle electrode is insulated, apart from its tip, and is placed, through the tympanic membrane, aseptically onto the promontory of the cochlea. It is kept in place by elastic hooked over the electrode holder. This stabilizes the electrode and maintains contact with the promontory (Fig. 4.3).

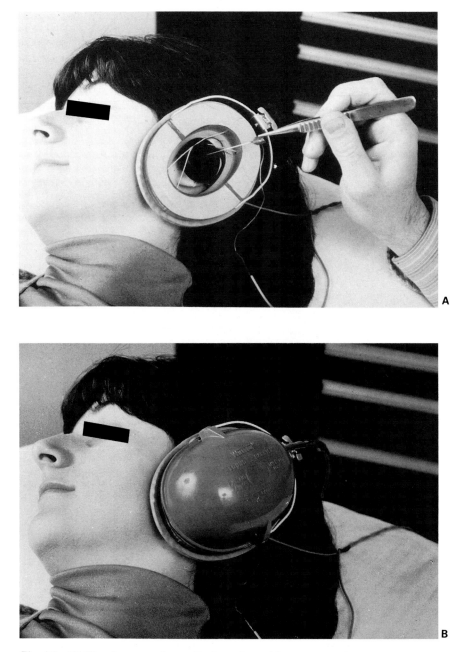

Fig. 4.3 (A) The placement of a needle electrode used in transtympanic electrocochleography. The earphone is held in position by the circumaural magnetic base so that it can be placed on the ear (B) after the electrode has been inserted.

The electrode is positioned midway between the tip of the malleus and the annulus of the tympanic membrane at the position of about 8 o'clock for the right ear, or 4 o'clock for the left ear. In this position, the electrode rests in front of and close to the round window niche. An operating microscope facilitates the accurate placement of the electrode. It should be noted that the closer the electrode is placed to the round window, the greater are the recorded potentials (Yoshie 1985).

Extratympanic ECochG has been recorded by implanting a needle electrode into the posterior meatal wall (Yoshie et al 1967, Elberling & Salomon 1971). In order to make the technique less invasive, various designs of non-traumatic surface electrodes in the form of a ball or wick attached to the wire have been placed on the eardrum (Cullen et al 1972, Khechinashvili & Kevanishvili 1974), or close to the annulus (Yoshie 1973, Coats 1974). Coats (1974) designed an atraumatic, external, auditory meatus electrode from a narrow strip of acetate, which he bent into 'V'-shape to provide the tension needed to maintain good contact. This electrode was inserted in a closed position with ear forceps. An insulated silver wire was connected to a 0.4 mm-diameter silver ball positioned at the tip of the electrode (Fig. 4.2). The contact point was located within 5 mm of the tympanic annulus in the area between 3 and 9 o'clock for the right ear. Singh et al (1980) obtained good-quality recordings by using an endomeatal silver/silver chloride electrode measuring $2 \times 1 \times 0.5$ mm and soldered to a very flexible wire. The electrode was attached with conductive electrode paste to the meatal wall close to the annulus at the level of about seven o'clock for the right ear or the equivalent 5 o'clock for the left ear.

The response amplitude depends upon the electrode position. The further away the electrode is from the annulus, the smaller is the compound action potential.

Both extratympanic and transtympanic methods require the expertise of an otologist in order to place the electrode safely in the right position, particularly when the needle has to be put through the eardrum. The extratympanic technique has the advantage that it is less invasive than the transtympanic ECochG. However, it may cause discomfort in a sensitive ear canal, and in small children it is not tolerated without general anaesthesia. The main response is at least 10 times greater than the potentials recorded by the extratympanic method. Moreover, the morphology of the waveform of the response is such that it is easier to identify the SP and AP components. Naturally, the signal-to-noise ratio is better when the transtympanic method is used as compared to the extratympanic method. Thus, the transtympanic technique has better sensitivity for threshold estimation. However, good morphology of SP and AP has been recorded in cases of mild hearing loss when an extratympanic electrode was used.

Ear-canal preparation to remove wax is usually necessary before introducing the electrode. A sterile needle electrode should be used, and an aseptic technique should be employed in placing the electrode. The transtympanic electrode usually can be stabilized in position better than extratympanic electrodes.

Anaesthesia for electrode placement

General anaesthesia is required in children in order to place the electrode. There is no evidence that general anaesthesia reduces the electro-cochleographic potentials. Inhalation anaesthesia is carried out with nitrous oxide, oxygen, and halothane.

Intramuscular injection of ketamine has been recommended for anaes-thesia in children under 3 years of age (Hutton 1981). Anaesthesia starts within a few minutes and lasts for about half an hour. If necessary, a second injection can be given.

ECochG under general anaesthesia in adults is very rarely indicated, and placement of both extratympanic and transtympanic electrodes can be tolerated without local anaesthesia on most occasions. Yoshie (1973) used a Japanese acupuncture needle as an electrode for his patients. The discomfort from the transtympanic method is comparable to that of a transcutaneous injection. For nervous patients, an anxiolytic dose of oral diazepam may be helpful. Also, it will improve the recording by reducing muscular activity and hence improving the signal-to-noise ratio.

A local injection of Xylocaine (0.1–0.2 ml) into the posterior meatal wall can also be used for anaesthesia. Spraying the eardrum with topical anaes-thetic, for example, Xylocaine (4%), probably has a placebo effect. Ion-tophoresis anaesthesia is thought to be effective for anaesthesia of the eardrum by some investigators. In this technique, an electric current is passed for about 11 minutes through an electrode immersed in a solution of Xylocaine (4%) with adrenaline and placed in the external auditory meatus.

Technical aspects of stimulation and recording

Brief-duration stimuli with short rise-fall times are essential to obtain a synchronized action potential from the cochlear nerve fibres which have a latency of only a few milliseconds. Clicks or very short tone bursts are most commonly used.

The commonest click stimulus is a square electrical impulse of 100 μs duration presented to an earphone or insert receiver. Tone bursts of several milliseconds, usually 4–20 ms in duration, can be used with short rise–fall times of 0.1–2 ms, depending on the frequency of the stimulus. Tone bursts of 2000 Hz and 1000 Hz should have rise–fall times of 1 ms and 2 ms, respectively. This can improve the frequency specificity of the AP when recorded close to the threshold. However, the main advantage of the tone bursts is in obtaining CM and SP. Simultaneous ipsilateral masking to obtain derived-responses can be used to get better, frequency-specific responses from the cochlea.

Electrodynamic headphones (for example, TDH-39 or TDH-49) can be placed on a circumaural ring such that the headphone does not touch the electrode. Alternatively, a loudspeaker can be positioned at a distance of 50 cm from the ear, and the stimuli delivered in the free field. In order to avoid electromagnetic artefacts contaminating this short latency response, a shielded headphone is desirable.

Monophasic or alternating polarity stimuli are presented at a repetition rate of 10/s. High-repetition rates of greater than 200/s can be used to adapt the AP, and provide a means of separating the non-adaptable SP from the SP/AP complex.

The number of sweeps per average ranges from 128 to 512, depending on conditions of recording and signal-to-noise ratio. Up to 1000 responses need to be averaged when an extratympanic electrode is used. Near-threshold replications of the response should be obtained to avoid false-positive errors, and at least two averages should be recorded and compared (Bell & Thornton 1988). The recommended recording bandwidth of the filters is 30–3000 Hz. The analysis window is 10–20 ms.

Computer manipulation techniques for separating CM, SP, and AP

Monophasic stimuli evoke a compound potential consisting of CM, SP and AP. The cochlear microphonic imitates the waveform of the acoustic stimulus, but the SP and AP have the same polarity irrespective of acoustic stimulus polarity. By using alternating-polarity stimuli, and storing the responses to condensation and rarefaction stimuli in separate buffers, the AP/SP complex can be separated from the CM. If the condensation stimuli are averaged separately into store A, and the opposite polarity rarefaction stimuli are averaged into store B, then the sum of the two responses (A+B) is a sum in which the CM has been cancelled, leaving the SP/AP complex (Fig. 4.4). Subtraction of one store from the other (A–B) leaves the CM and cancels the SP/AP complex.

The SP can be separated from the AP by obtaining a response to a fast-repetition rate of 200 stimuli/s, which adapts the AP to practically zero, but leaves the SP unchanged (see Fig. 3.9). Having obtained the SP from the high-repetition rate response, one may then subtract it from the slow-repetition rate response to give the AP alone.

NORMATIVE CHARACTERISTICS OF ECochG

A full picture of cochlear function is based upon the assessment of all three components, CM, SP, and AP. The waveform morphology, the amplitudes of the components, and the latency of AP are used as parameters of ECochG.

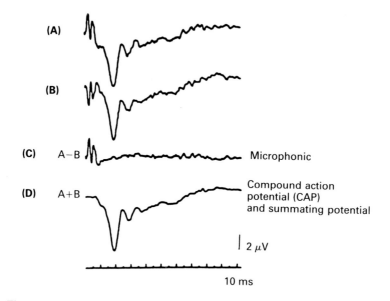

Fig. 4.4 Computer manipulation techniques for separating the CM and SP/AP complex. (**A**) The recorded waveform using a condensation click and CM, SP, and CAP. (**B**) A second recorded waveform using a rarefaction click. (**C**) The result of subtracting B from A. Only the antiphasic CM is left; the CAP and SP are cancelled. (**D**) The result of adding A and B. The antiphasic CM is cancelled, and the SP/CAP complex remains.

In the succeeding sections, the cochlear microphonic (CM), the summating potential (SP), and the action potential (AP) are dealt with separately. In practice, of course, these responses arrive overlapping in time and have to be separated.

This separation may be achieved by a method based on the following properties of these responses: (a) The CM follows the polarity of the stimulus; (b) the AP remains the same independently of stimulus polarity; (c) the SP does not adapt to high stimulation rates; and (d) the AP does adapt to high stimulation rates.

Either by altering the click-stimulus polarity or by averaging separately the responses to condensation and rarefaction clicks, the CM can be eliminated. In the former case, it is automatically cancelled in computing the average, as for each pair of sweeps the CM appears with opposite polarities. In the latter case, the two waveforms may be added together in order to cancel the CM and leave the SP/AP complex. If separate averages of condensation and rarefaction clicks have been taken, then the subtraction of one waveform from the other will cancel the SP/AP complex and yield the CM on its own (Fig. 4.4).

Having removed the CM by one of the methods described above, one may then repeat the test, using a click-stimulus rate of around 100/s. This will adapt the AP to virtually zero and leave the SP in the waveform. This waveform may then be subtracted from the SP/AP-complex waveform to give the AP alone. In this way, all these three components may be isolated and their properties studied individually.

Cochlear microphonic (CM)

The cochlear microphonic (CM) is generated by the hair cells and reflects the mechano-electrical transduction process in the cochlea. Von Békésy (1960) showed that the CM is proportional to the displacement of the normal cochlear partition. However, one should bear in mind that the CM, as recorded by a transtympanic electrode, represents a spatial average, and predominant contributions come from the basal turn, irrespective of the stimulus frequency. The experiments of Dallos (1976) have shown that the outer hair cells (OHC) are 30–40 dB more sensitive than the inner hair cells (IHC). It was found that the contribution to the CM by the IHC is, at most, one-tenth of the contribution from the OHC (Davis et al 1958, Dallos & Wang 1974, Dallos 1976). Dallos (1976) also showed that at high-stimulus levels the CM exhibits non-linearity. He concluded that at low intensities (fewer than 50 dB SPL) the CM, produced by OHC, is proportional to the displacement of the cochlear partition. But at higher intensities the CM, produced by IHC, is proportional to the velocity of the partition (Dallos 1973).

Waveform

The CM can be obtained in response to a monophasic polarity click. However, the best responses are obtained from tone-burst stimulation.

Clinical use of the CM waveform is limited, as its amplitude varies greatly among subjects. The electromagnetic and acoustic microphonic effects of the electrode itself may be distinguished from genuine CM only by the characteristics of the amplitude–intensity function. At low levels, all signals have a linear function. However, as the level is increased, the acoustic microphonic and other artefactual responses continue to increase with stimulus intensity, whereas the true CM is limited and then shows a decrease in amplitude at stimulus levels of 80–90 dBnHL.

Amplitude and intensity–amplitude relationship

The relatively small amplitude of the CM and its large variation among subjects imposes limitations on the use of quantitative measurements of CM as a diagnostic parameter (Hoke 1976).

The CM detection threshold in the normal ear is about 50 dBnHL at 4000 Hz when using 4-ms-duration tone bursts with a rise-fall time of 0.1 ms (Kumagami et al 1982).

Aran & Charlet de Sauvage (1976) showed that the distribution of CM amplitudes evoked by click stimuli in a population of normal ears is

Gaussian. In recording from the promontory at 95 dBnHL, the mean amplitude was 10.9 μV with a standard deviation of 7.4 μV.

Non-linearities in the hydrodynamics of the inner ear and in mechano-electrical transduction have a significant effect on both the amplitude and phase of the CM. There is a large variability in these non-linear effects among subjects (Hoke 1976), and this limits the clinical quantitative use of this parameter.

Summating potential (SP)

When the CM is 'stripped' away from the ECochG recording, one sees a step-like, direct-current voltage, which, in normal subjects, is identifiable as a negative trough on the limb of the compound AP (Fig. 4.5). This is called the summating potential (SP). The SP is a DC response of the cochlea to acoustic stimuli, and this phenomenon obviously is non-linear. The SP is thought to be a distortion product of the hair-cell transduction process; it is generated when the membrane changes its electrical resistance as the basilar membrane is displaced.

Experimental SP recordings with electrodes in the scala vestibuli (SV) and scala tympani (ST) give SPs of differing magnitudes and polarities (Dallos et al 1972, Dallos 1976).

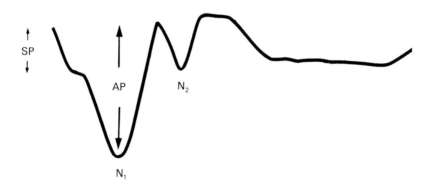

Fig. 4.5 The summating potential in the SP/AP complex. The SP is most clearly seen as a negative step preceding the AP.

SP waveform

The SP can be seen in a click-evoked response (Fig. 4.6), but better responses are obtained from tone-burst stimulation, and these are of greater magnitude when recorded by the transtympanic method than with the extratympanic method. Eggermont (1976) used tone bursts of 2000, 4000, and 8000 Hz with rise–fall times of 2 periods and a plateau duration of at least

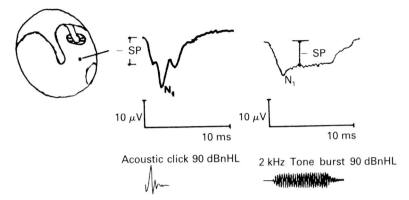

Fig. 4.6 The SP in the SP/AP complex in response to click- and tone-burst stimuli. The SP duration approximates to the duration of the tone burst. Note the position of the transtympanic electrode in relation to the ossicles and the round window.

4 ms. The SP duration approximates to the duration of the tone burst. The SP in a man, when recorded from the promontory, is usually a negative deflection (SP−) which appears on the leading part of the AP. However, very occasionally, a positive deflection (SP+) can be recorded in response to stimulation with high-frequency, high-intensity tone bursts, and this may revert to the normal negative polarity at lower intensities (Eggermont 1976). The polarity of the SP is usually negative for all frequencies except those at 8000 Hz or above, as shown in Figures 4.7 and 4.8 (Dauman et al 1986; Yoshie 1985).

Some difficulty in identification of the SP in the compound action potential may occur. High-repetition stimulation of 200/s can be applied in order to adapt the neurogenic AP component. A rapid indication of the SP component can be made by comparing electrocochleographic response at the usual slow-repetition rate of 10/s with the fast-repetition rate of 200/s.

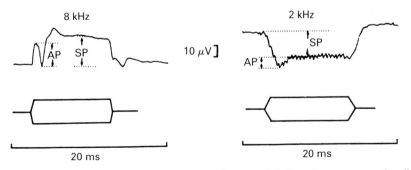

Fig. 4.7 Polarity of the SP is usually negative when recorded from the promontory for all frequencies except 8000 Hz or above. (Reproduced with permission from Dauman R et al 1986.)

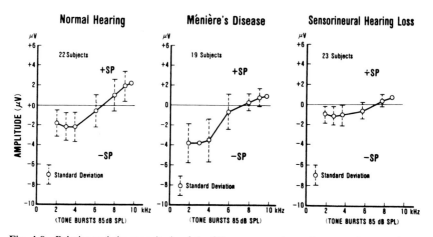

Fig. 4.8 Polarity and the magnitude of the SP versus tone-burst frequency in normal subjects, those with Ménière's disease, and those with sensorineural hearing loss. (Reproduced with permission from Yoshie N 1985.)

It is advisable to place the electrode close to the round window, in order to avoid the isopotential line between the oval and round windows.

Amplitude and intensity–amplitude relationship

If the threshold of the SP is defined as the intensity at which the SP amplitude is equal to 0.1 μV, then, in normal subjects, the threshold is about 50 dBnHL. The amplitude at a particular stimulus intensity shows a considerable variation among subjects. This could be due to slight variations in electrode position as well as to variations in the contact impedance of the needle electrode. Using 4-ms-duration tone bursts of 2000 Hz at 85 dBnHL, Eggermont (1976) recorded SPs with amplitudes ranging from 0.3 to 6.0 μV.

In normal cochleae undergoing tone-burst stimulation, the mean amplitude of the SP increases with rising frequencies from 2000 to 4000 Hz, according to Yoshie (1985). The slope of the intensity–amplitude function of the SP is similar to the slope of the CM.

SP/AP ratio

Because the amplitude variability of both SP and AP may be due, in large part, to variations in electrode location and electrode impedance, a relative value of the ratio of SP/AP has been suggested (Gibson et al 1983).

In normal ears, the SP/AP ratio increases with the stimulus intensity to about 30% when using tone bursts of 2000 Hz at 85 dBnHL. When tone bursts of several milliseconds were used, the SP measured from the zero baseline to around the middle of the analysis window on the screen. The

AP is measured between the SP baseline and the peak of the AP. When a click stimulus at 100 dBnHL was used, the mean SP/AP value was reported to be 25% with a standard deviation of 14% (Gibson et al 1983) (see Fig. 4.5 and 4.6).

The changes in SP/AP ratio have been observed as a function of tone-burst frequency in normal ears and were largest for stimuli in the 2000–4000 Hz region. The SP/AP ratio at 6000–8000 Hz is highly variable among subjects and, therefore, clinically less useful (Ohashi et al 1985).

Stimulus–repetition rates of more than 12/s decrease the AP amplitude, and, consequently, increase the SP/AP ratio.

Recording from the external auditory meatus has been advocated by several investigators (Coats 1986, Mason et al 1980). Ferraro et al (1985) reported mean SP/AP values in the normal population to be 0.28, with less than 6% of the values being greater than 0.50.

The compound action potential

The compound action potential (CAP) represents the synchronized response of many neurones. Broad-band clicks or high-level tone bursts produce the CAP.

Waveform

The CAP waveform at high intensities is seen as a series of two (sometimes three) negative peaks, which are labelled N1 and N2 (Fig. 4.9). The series of peaks represents the convolution of a sequence of responses along the basilar membrane.

The CAP response contributions from different areas of the basilar membrane have been studied by using various stimuli and by simultaneously restricting response from unwanted areas by employing masking techniques (Eggermont et al 1976a, 1976b; Elberling 1976; Zerlin & Nauton 1976). Analysis of AP is derived from the shape of AP. The width of the narrow-band contributions reflects the synchronization, which is better at higher frequencies when the basal turn of the cochlea is stimulated, and the AP is narrower. The delayed latency of AP for lower frequencies reflects the travelling wave velocity along the basilar membrane and the apical shift in the cochlea of the AP response.

Amplitude and intensity–amplitude relationship

The amplitude of N1, measured from the baseline to its negative peak, depends on the stimulus intensity. In tone-burst stimulation, as the frequency decreases, the amplitude gets smaller. For example, when stimulated at 90 dBnHL, the AP amplitude changes from 25 μV, in response to 4000-Hz tone bursts, to 15.6 μV, when 2000-Hz tone bursts are used.

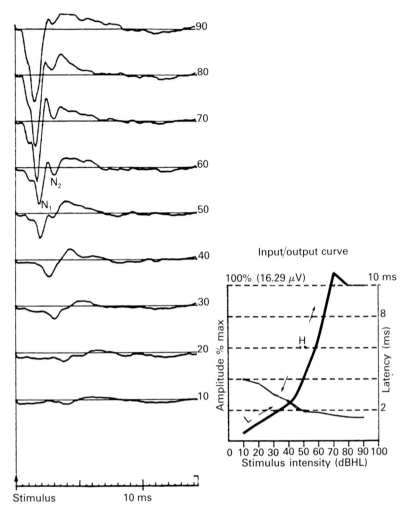

Fig. 4.9 The CAP at different click intensities and the amplitude and latency input/output curves in a patient with normal hearing. Note the L and H segments of the curve and the waveforms, which are predominantly monophasic at the high intensities and become more biphasic as the intensity is reduced. Note that here, and in some subsequent figures, the SP appears to be delayed and have a latency of about 0.4 ms. However, this reflects the filter propagation delay discussed in Chapter 3.

The relationship between stimulus intensity and response amplitude is called the input/output (I/O) function of the AP. A normal result is shown in Figure 4.9. With click stimulation, the I/O function contains a low slope (L) section in its response to the lower intensity stimuli, and a steeper section of high slope (H) in response to signals of about 50 dBnHL and higher. The transition between these two slope sections can vary but is often reflected as a new point.

The most reasonable explanation for the L and H sections is the 'recruiting' argument, which is that at low intensities the finely tuned VIIIth nerve fibres are being stimulated. As the stimulus is increased at low intensities, only a few fibres are involved, and the I/O function grows slowly. However, once an intensity of about 50 or 60 dBnHL is reached, the signal can stimulate the low-frequency 'tails' of the high-frequency fibres (see Fig. 2.4). Suddenly, a large number of fibres are 'recruited' and contribute towards the response, giving a steeper slope to the I/O function. This explains the difference in the L and H slope sections and is consistent with the results found in patients who show classical 'recruitment'. In these cases, the I/O function is predominantly the high-frequency slope portion of the normal curve (see Fig. 4.10).

At the transition between the H and L curves, both the short latency (H response) and the longer latency (L response) may be present, giving rise

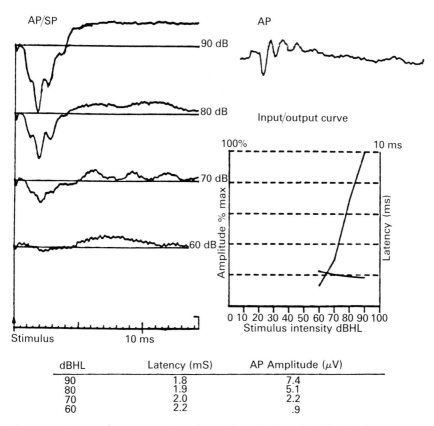

dBHL	Latency (mS)	AP Amplitude (μV)
90	1.8	7.4
80	1.9	5.1
70	2.0	2.2
60	2.2	.9

Fig. 4.10   The input/output curve in patient with recruiting cochlear hearing loss (Ménière's disease). Note that there is only the steep H slope part of the I/O function. The waveforms on the left are AP/SP complexes, showing the broad shape often seen in Ménière's disease. The waveform on the right is the 90-dB response with the SP removed. This shows a narrow AP, demonstrating that the broadening is due to the SP.

to a double-peaked response waveform. When the intensity–amplitude function is evaluated, the amplitude of the AP can be expressed as a percentage of the maximum response, usually in response to signals of about 90 dBnHL.

In summary, it is evident that at high-stimulus intensities, the main CAP contribution is from the neurones innervating the basal part of the cochlea. Poor synchronization of the later-activated neurones results in out-of-phase, partial self-cancellation of the AP contributions from more apical parts of the cochlea.

Latency and intensity–latency relationship

In near-threshold stimulation, the latency of the CAP increases as the frequency of a tone-burst stimulus decreases, as a result of apical shift of response initiation on the basilar membrane.

The latency is a function of stimulus intensity, and it gets shorter with increasing stimulus intensity. The plotted curve of intensity–latency function can be, accordingly, divided into L-, and H-response segments. The AP latencies in response to low-intensity clicks or L-responses vary from 2 to 5 ms, and the latencies at the higher intensities of an H-response are considerably shorter, varying in a narrower range between 1.5 and 2.0 ms. In the human cochlea, there is a sudden shortening in latency at intensities between 60 and 70 dBnHL.

Frequency selectivity

Each neurone in the cochlear nerve responds best at a particular stimulus frequency known as its characteristic frequency (CF). Thus, tone bursts, at low intensity, evoke an AP which is generated by synchronous activity in a limited number of neurones which have similar CFs. Methods of measuring the frequency-selectivity function have been described by Eggermont (1977) and by Harrison & Aran (1982) (Fig. 4.11). These methods are based on tone-suppression paradigms which involve masking techniques and which have enabled the measurement of parameters such as the CF and the width of the tuning curve corresponding to a 50% reduction in AP amplitude. The measurement of these 'physiologic tuning curves' in man and the effects of pathologies on the width of the tuning curves have been demonstrated (Harrison & Aran 1982). In sensorineural hearing loss, the tuning curve was much wider than in normal subjects and hence the frequency selectivity function was degraded.

Adaptation function

Spoor et al (1976) showed that the CAP amplitude decays exponentially during the first five stimulus presentations, and that thereafter it has an approximately constant amplitude.

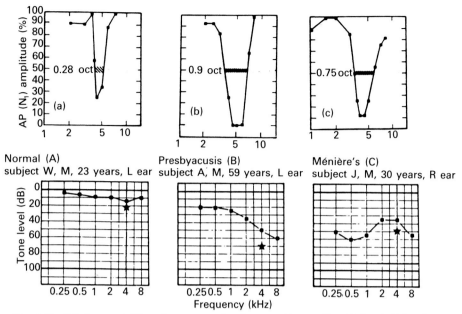

Fig. 4.11 (**A**) A normal AP tuning curve and audiogram. Abnormally wide bandwidths of the AP tuning curve in two kinds of cochlear hearing loss: (**B**) in presbyacusis and (**C**) in Ménière's disease. (Reproduced with permission from Harrison R V & Aran J-M 1982.)

FACTORS INFLUENCING NORMAL ECochG

Age

It has been reported that with increasing age, the CM decreases (Aran & Charlet de Sauvage 1976). This is probably due to OHC depletion (Soucek 1989).

Sedatives and anaesthetics

General anaesthesia does not have a direct effect on the potentials generated in the cochlea. The AP latencies of those subjects tested under general anaesthesia fall within the range of those who did not require the anaesthetic.

Stimulation rate

Increase in stimulation rate has a noticeable effect on the amplitude and latency of the AP. For 4000-Hz tone bursts at 95 dBnHL, changes in inter-stimulus interval from 128 to 16 ms caused a decrease in AP amplitude of nearly 50%, and the latency was prolonged by 0.4 ms (Spoor et al 1976).

FREQUENCY SPECIFICITY OF ECochG

In the normal cochlea, the N1 response to a click originates predominantly in the basal turn. If N1 is detected within 10 dBnHL and the latency is normal, then the audiogram is normal in the 2000–4000 Hz region.

At higher intensities, the excitation pattern in the cochlea widens, as it is only near the threshold that any frequency specificity can be obtained.

The frequency specificity of a stimulus is determined by its spectrum. The longer the duration of a tone burst, the more frequency-specific it becomes. However, it is a general rule in evoked-response work that frequency-specific stimuli do not necessarily produce frequency-specific responses, and so care must be taken in interpreting the results obtained with tone bursts.

Eggermont (1979) has described a method of measuring the frequency specificity of electrocochleographic responses in man. He recorded derived or narrow-band action potentials (NAP), as shown in Figure 4.12. He then mapped the NAP amplitudes as a function of the central frequency for the narrow band and compared the results obtained for different types of

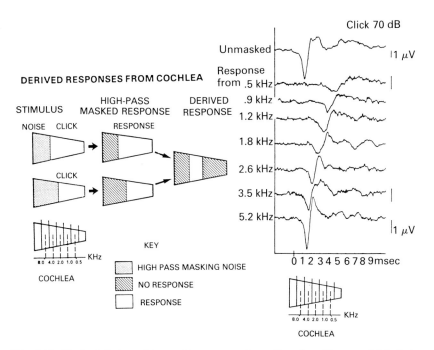

Fig. 4.12 Derived electrocochleographic responses (recordings from Eggermont J J et al 1976). The top trace is the compound action potential (CAP) in response to a click. The derived-responses are shown with the centre frequency of the derived band as a parameter. The low-frequency responses are broader and have longer latencies than do the CAP or the high-frequency derived-responses. This is a reflection of the basilar membrane travelling wave propagation.

stimuli. As expected, a click stimulus produced a broad spectrum in the evoked response, and a 2000-Hz tone burst produced a narrower spectrum. However, the 2000-Hz tone-burst spectrum estimated from response measurement was considerably wider than the acoustical spectrum of the tone burst. At 70 dBnHL the 2000-Hz tone burst produced the spectral limits of the response, ranging from about 900 to 5500 Hz. Only at low intensity levels did the excitation spectrum correspond to the acoustic spectrum.

This implies that tone-burst stimuli may be used to obtain frequency-specific thresholds if the difference between electrophysiologic and subjective thresholds is not large and if there are no problems of effective stimulation level caused by 'recruiting' hearing pathologies.

In general, responses to lower-frequency stimuli at 1000 Hz and 500 Hz give inadequate results because of the broadening and reduced amplitude of N1 as a result of poor synchronization further apically along the basilar membrane.

ECochG audiometry with tone bursts does not guarantee frequency specificity even in the middle- and high-range audiometric frequencies. But it is possible to estimate frequency-specific thresholds by using high-pass masking techniques to obtain derived narrow-band AP (NAP).

The accuracy of frequency specificity in the presence of severe hearing loss or high-frequency hearing loss with a steep audiometric slope is not well quantified. However, by using masking procedures in the same ear, one can estimate such audiograms (Eggermont 1979).

THRESHOLD ESTIMATION

ECochG can be done non-invasively, with the electrode in the external meatus. The amplitude is decreased by a factor which varies among patients, but which is, roughly, at least 10–20 times (Mori et al 1982). This recording site reduces the response's audiometric sensitivity, but by how much is unclear. There is also a considerable variation in the clarity and reliability of the meatal recordings obtained by different investigators. Simmons (1976) compared AP thresholds in normal subjects for three electrode locations. He found that the transtympanic electrode, the needle electrode placed immediately beside the annulus, and the saline wick electrode placed close to the annulus were capable of giving threshold or near-threshold N1 responses, but only the promontory method did so consistently, as compared to other methods which had considerable scatter.

Experience indicates that the transtympanic ECochG has very good sensitivity for threshold estimation when click- or tone-burst stimuli at frequencies above 2000 Hz are used (Ryerson & Beagley 1981), and that the threshold sensitivity in normal subjects is about 10 dB (Fig. 4.5). At lower frequencies the accuracy is degraded (Davis 1981). However, there are reports of satisfactory responses using even 500-Hz tone-burst stimuli (Eggermont et al 1976).

5. ECochG in hearing disorders

ECochG IN CONDUCTIVE HEARING LOSS

Pathophysiology

Hearing levels are elevated in patients with conductive hearing loss due to affected sound transmission and reduction of the stimulus energy reaching the cochlea. Responses from such patients, will correspond to normative ECochG responses at the appropriate sensation level.

Effect of conductive-type hearing loss

Compared to normal values, the mean CM and SP amplitudes decrease with increasing hearing loss. The AP has a normal pattern but with decreased amplitude. The latencies are prolonged and correspond proportionally to the sensation level of the stimulus. Note that in cases of middle ear effusion, the normal practice is, preceding ECochG, to carry out a myringotomy and aspirate the fluid.

Hearing loss estimation

The difference between normal threshold and a patient's estimated threshold indicates the hearing loss. ECochG is poor at estimating hearing levels for low frequencies.

Prolongation of the AP latency and the intensity–latency function suggests a conductive hearing loss although it is not diagnostic.

Differentiating between conductive and cochlear losses

The AP latency should be measured at several intensities. If the curve thus obtained follows the shape of the normal latency by intensity function but is displaced to higher intensity values, then the loss is conductive and may be estimated from the average displacement. A cochlear 'recruiting' impairment gives 'displaced' values at lower intensities, but these values are identical to or approach normal ones at higher intensities (see p. 68).

Bone-conduction electrocochleography has been used to measure air–bone gaps, but because of the technical problems created by the electromagnetic artefact from a normal bone conductor, the technique is not widely used.

ECochG IN COCHLEAR HEARING LOSS

Pathophysiology of electrocochleographic responses

The damage to the hair cells that occurs in cochlear hearing loss is associated with a reduction of CM (Ramsden et al 1980, Keen & Graham 1984) and also SP.

If the hair cells in the basal turn are damaged, the contribution from the apical region may become dominant. This results in a prolongation of the latency of the AP due to travelling wave delay. As the synchrony is poorer in the apical region, the waveform may be broader. The waveform of the AP will be, consequently, abnormal. In moderate sensory hearing loss, in which only the outer hair cells have been damaged, the AP can be almost normal for high-intensity stimuli (Aran 1971). Small increments in stimulus intensity may result in inadequate response, manifested in recruitment and abnormal intensity–amplitude function. Cochlear lesions may also affect the tuning mechanism of the cochlea, and result in an abnormal frequency-selectivity function.

Cochlear microphonic

The CM can be recorded for both click and tone-burst stimuli. It is assumed that in patients with cochlear hearing loss and recruitment, there is hair cell loss. In those patients, the CM in response to high-intensity clicks is considerably smaller than in normal subjects. In the absence of the AP, CMs recorded in patients with severe hearing loss should be interpreted very carefully, as they may be indistinguishable from electromagnetic artefacts (see p. 51).

Various cochlear pathologies show considerable variation in the degree of hair cell loss. Moreover, the activity of the remaining hair cells, as represented by the CM, can vary a great deal; so, quantitative estimates are unreliable.

Table 4.1 CM amplitude at 95 dBnHL as a function of AP threshold

AP threshold (dBnHL)	CM amplitude (μV): Mean	SD
0–20	10.9	7.4
20–40	6.05	7.2
40–60	4.8	3.54
60–80	4.85	5.05
80–95	1.53	1.61

In general, the amplitude of the CM gets smaller with increasing hearing loss. A representative example from Aran & Charlet de Sauvage (1976) shows CM amplitude at click stimulus intensity of 95 dBnHL as a function of the AP threshold (Table 4.1).

Summating potential

In cochlear hearing loss due to ototoxic drugs, noise, asphyxia, etc., the SP amplitude is significantly smaller than that recorded in normal subjects (Yoshie 1985). This small amplitude is attributed to hair cell loss and varies from 0 to 1 μV in response to an 80–90 dBnHL stimulus. The amplitude of the SP varies in individuals with the same hearing loss, and depends on the type of the lesion. The intensity–amplitude curves of the SP were below normal in 79% of the cases studied by Ohashi & Yoshie (1985).

The SP/AP ratio is also smaller in patients suffering cochlear hearing loss than in normal subjects.

Action potential

AP Waveform in cochlear hearing loss

Different waveform patterns at high-intensity stimulation have been recorded in pathological conditions; these have been described as normal, recruiting, abnormally broad, dissociated, and less clearly defined, abnormally shaped responses (Aran 1973) (Fig. 5.1, Fig. 5.5).

The shape of the normal I/O function has been explained in Chapter 4. The waveforms associated with a normal I/O function are essentially 'monophasic' at high intensities. That is, the positive peak following N1 does not overshoot the baseline or, at least, does not exceed it by a great deal. At lower intensities the waveform is 'biphasic'.

However, in classical recruiting cases the waveform remains 'biphasic' at high-intensity levels. Evans (1975) has explained this in terms of damage to hair cell tuning. The shape of the I/O function is that of the H section, as explained in Chapter 4.

A broad SP/AP complex may be recorded in pathologies such as Ménière's disease, acoustic neurinoma, and high-frequency sensorineural hearing loss (Fig. 5.5). However, the reasons for such a response can be different.

In Ménière's disease, the AP can be normal, but the SP is large and of an abnormal duration, presumably because of the abnormal cochlear pressures. Thus, the SP/AP complex is broad, entirely as a result of the SP, as shown in Figure 3.9(a).

In acoustic neurinomas and, indeed, in some cases of high-frequency sensorineural hearing loss, the SP/AP complex is broad as a result of an abnormally broad AP (Fig. 5.5). This occurs in the high-frequency loss case because a broad AP is generated by the responding low-frequency fibres.

In the case of acoustic neurinoma, it is most likely that desynchronization of the unit APs is the cause. These cases illustrate the occasional need to examine the SP and AP components separately.

The dissociated response is encountered in high-frequency hearing loss with a steep slope (Fig. 5.1). The dissociated response is characterized by a sudden increase in latency as the intensity decreases. This occurs in high-frequency hearing loss cases, because a short-latency response from the high-frequency fibres can be recorded only at high intensities. As the in-

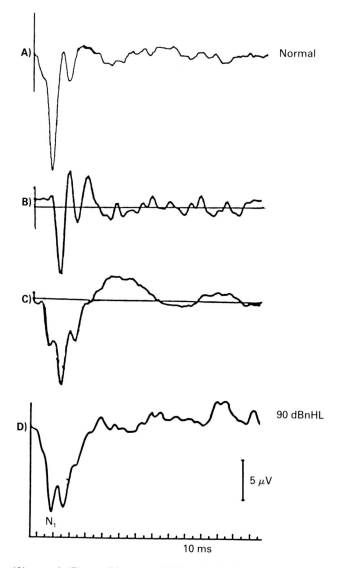

Fig. 5.1 (**A**) normal; (**B**) recruiting type; (**C**) broad; (**D**) dissociated.

tensity is reduced, there comes a point at which the short-latency response from the high-frequency fibres becomes very small, and the response from the lower-frequency fibres, which, in this case, have better thresholds, predominates. Because of the travelling wave delay, the low-frequency response has a longer latency, and so a 'step' in the latency I/O function can be seen. Often, at the transition level, we find a double-peaked response in which both the high- and low-frequency responses occur.

Amplitude and latency input/output functions

In 'recruiting' cochlear lesions, there is an elevated threshold (often of the order of 40–50 dB HTL), and the latency at the threshold is shorter than normal, as it is due to the high-frequency fibres and is associated with the H section of the amplitude I/O function (see p. 56 and Fig. 4.9). The amplitude then increases with the increase in stimulus intensity at a greater rate than normal and has a near normal value at high intensities (Fig. 5.2). In high-frequency hearing loss cases, the 'dissociated' response is often found.

Frequency-selectivity function .

The AP may be used to estimate frequency selectivity (see Chapter 4), and Harrison & Aran (1982) have reported abnormalities in various pathologies. Figure 4.10 shows the audiograms and tuning curves for a normal subject, a patient with presbyacusis, and one with Ménière's disease. The width of the 'tuning curve' is greatly increased in the pathological cases. Frequency selectivity can be impaired in various cochlear pathologies and can occur with minor audiometric deficit.

ECochG IN MÉNIÈRE'S DISEASE

Pathophysiology

Endolymphatic hydrops causes distension of the membranous labyrinthine spaces and is thought to be a pathological feature of Ménière's disease (Hallpike & Cairns 1938, Schuknecht 1982, Dohlmann 1983, Paparella 1985). Endolymphatic hydrops is likely to affect the static displacement of the cochlear partition. Improvement of the audiometric threshold and reduction of the SP and of the SP/AP ratio under the influence of osmotic, dehydrating agents, such as glycerol or manitol, has been demonstrated (Moffat et al 1978, Morrison et al 1980, Coats & Alford 1981). ECochG has also been used in evaluating decompression surgery (Booth 1980).

Hydrops can lead to secondary pathological changes of the hair cells and, hence, give rise to a recruiting pattern in the intensity–amplitude function and to a deterioration in the frequency-selectivity function.

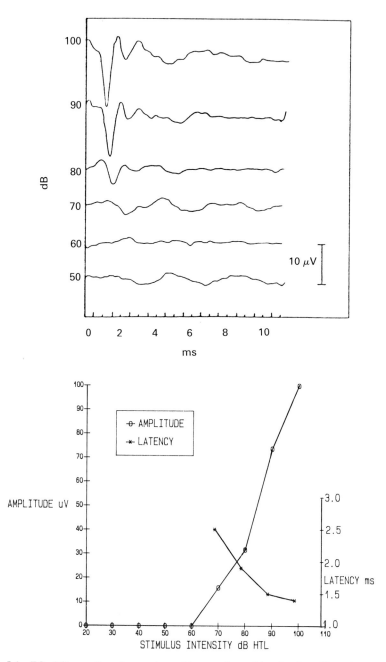

Fig. 5.2 ECochG recordings in a patient with sensorineural hearing loss. Note the small SP. The latency and amplitude are normal at high intensities, and the I/O curve is of a recruiting type.

Cochlear microphonic

It has been shown that in patients with Ménière's disease the CM amplitude shows no significant difference from normal values for a 95 dBnHL click. However, when comparing the CM of patients with Ménière's disease (mean = 4.76 μV; SD = 3.53 μV) with the CM in patients with cochlear hearing loss (assumed hair cell loss) (mean = 2.45 μV; SD = 2.29 μV), there was a significant difference in the response to 95 dBnHL clicks (Aran & Charlet de Sauvage 1976).

The presence of a recordable CM implies at least a functional population of hair cells.

The CM detection threshold in Ménière' disease patients who have only a mild hearing loss is almost the same as in normal subjects. However, the detection threshold increases with the degree of hearing loss.

The CM threshold in patients with fluctuating hearing losses was better than in patients who had minimal or no fluctuation of the hearing level, although the pure-tone audiograms were similar (Kumagami et al 1982).

Summating potential

With click stimuli, SP and AP components appear combined in the ECochG response in the form of CAP. When using tone bursts, one finds the components usually much easier to distinguish and separate. An enhanced SP has been described in Ménière's disease, with the largest amplitudes being given by tone bursts at 1000 Hz and 2000 Hz, as compared with 4000- and 8000-Hz tone bursts or broad-band clicks (Fig. 5.3).

A wide variation in SP amplitudes, with a mean amplitude of 2.5 μV in response to 2000-Hz tone bursts at 85 dBnHL, has been recorded by Eggermont (1976) and Eggermont et al (1980). These values are similar to those of normal subjects, whereas the average hearing threshold was 40 dBnHL, and the AP thresholds were elevated.

The intensity–amplitude function for click stimulation in Ménière's disease patients with mild, fluctuating, and moderate hearing levels is almost the same as in normal subjects, but for those with mild and fluctuating losses the SP is greater than normal for tone burst stimulation at 80 and 90 dBnHL (Kumagami et al 1982). It has been assumed that the increase in SP may be related to endolymphatic hydrops.

SP/AP ratio

The SP/AP ratio in response to click stimuli gives a better representation of any abnormality than does the absolute amplitude of the SP itself (Fig. 5.4), because it reduces the variability among subjects. The SP/AP ratio is not used for tone bursts below 2000 Hz, because the AP is poorly recorded from the more apical region.

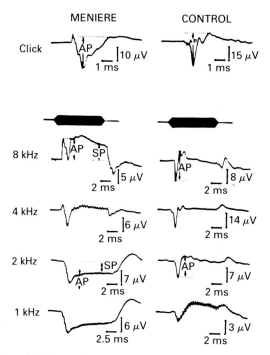

Fig. 5.3 An enhanced SP in Ménière's disease, with the largest amplitudes being produced by tone bursts at 1000 and 2000 Hz, as compared with tone bursts at 4000 and 8000 Hz or with clicks. (From Dauman et al 1988, with permission.)

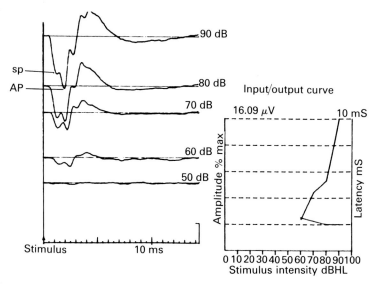

Fig. 5.4 Electrocochleogram of a patient with Ménière's disease. Note the enhanced SP (SP/AP ratio of greater than 50%) and a steep recruiting type I/O curve.

In a Ménière's disease group, both SP amplitude and SP/AP ratio were measured as a function of stimulus intensity for 4000-Hz tone bursts. The SP amplitude–intensity curves were within the normal range in 58% of cases, whilst the SP/AP ratio amplitude–intensity curves were greater than normal in 75% of cases (Ohashi et al 1985).

The mean value of the SP/AP ratio in Ménière's disease patients with mild hearing loss is 0.3, which is close to that of normal subjects. However, in patients with both fluctuating and non-fluctuating degrees of moderate hearing loss, the SP/AP mean values were greater than 0.4, according to Kumagami et al (1982).

Gibson et al (1983) found that with hearing levels below 40 dB no obvious difference was apparent in SP/AP ratio between Ménière's disease patients and normal subjects. Above 40 dB, however, a clear separation appeared between Ménière's disease patients and patients with sensory hearing loss. In the sensory group, the amplitudes of both SP and AP declined with increasing hearing loss. In the Ménière's group, the amplitude of the AP declined similarly, but the SP remained relatively unchanged. In the early stages of Ménière's disease, one can assume that the SP normally generated in cochleae arises from a non-linearity of the basilar membrane response. However, in later stages of Ménière's disease, where the moderate hearing loss manifests itself, Gibson et al (1983) have suggested that, although there is hair cell loss, asymmetry of the basilar membrane, as a result of endo-lymphatic hydrops, may be responsible for the generation of greater SP potentials.

Ferraro et al (1985) studied the SP/AP ratio, recorded with an endomeatal electrode, in relation to clinical symptoms. All the subjects who were totally asymptomatic on the day of testing had normal ECochG. When symptoms were present, the combination of hearing loss and a feeling of fullness or pressure was the strongest predictor of an enlarged SP/AP ratio of more than 0.5.

Action potential

Waveform

A proportion of patients with Ménière's disease exhibit an enlarged, negative SP, which is apparent in a broadening of the AP/SP complex.

Amplitude and latency input/output functions

The amplitude and latency I/O functions are similar to those found in cochlear hearing loss (see Fig. 5.4).

ECochG IN ACOUSTIC TUMOURS

Pathophysiology

ECochG assesses the state of hearing at the peripheral site of the internal auditory meatus (IAM), but does not reflect subsequent events occurring further along the nerve and the auditory pathway. It is thought that acoustic tumours produce hearing loss by damaging the cochlea, often by interfering with the blood supply.

Cochlear microphonic

Preservation of a good cochlear microphonic potential has been observed in acoustic tumours (Morrison et al 1976), and has been considered to be one of the diagnostic criteria. Such a response is associated with more medially located tumours.

Summating potential

In acoustic tumours that cause a high-frequency hearing loss of greater than 50 dBnHL, there is a noticeable decrease in SP, and this decrease is more marked the higher the stimulus frequency. In general, the median values of the SP in acoustic tumours are lower than in Ménière's disease (Eggermont et al 1980).

There is a wide variation in SP/AP ratio in acoustic tumours, ranging both below and above the normal values, depending on the pathological involvement of the hair cells and the cochlear nerve. The SP/AP ratio values fall within the normal range in about one-third of all acoustic tumours (Yoshie 1985). In some cases, developing secondary endolymphatic hydrops may contribute to enhanced SP values and greater than normal SP/AP values.

Action potential

Waveform

It has been reported that VIIIth nerve tumours cause abnormally broad AP waveforms of more than 4 ms when measured at the baseline (Fig. 5.5). However, broad AP waveforms also occur in various pathologies, including Ménière's disease, as a result of the abnormal SP (Gibson & Beagley 1976, Gibson et al 1977, Morrison et al 1976; Brackmann & Selters 1976; Portmann & Aran 1972). In order to avoid the confounding effect of SP, the wave form width was measured at about one-third of the AP amplitude, in response to a tone burst of 4 ms duration. A critical appraisal of this parameter, in acoustic tumours, showed that only about 30% of cases were outside the normal range (Eggermont et al 1980).

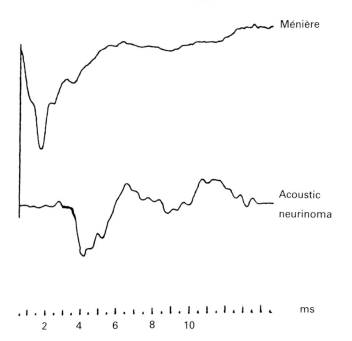

Ménière

Acoustic
neurinoma

2   4   6   8   10   ms

Fig. 5.5 ECochG waveform in an acoustic neuroma case (the bottom trace), with high frequency hearing loss on the audiogram. The waveform is broad and less well-formed than normal.

In general, the AP waveform depends on stimulus frequency, stimulus intensity, audiometric contour (see p. 65), and pathology. A broad waveform can result from a large negative SP, high-frequency hearing loss, or poor synchrony of the response.

Eggermont et al (1980), using 2000-, 4000-, and 8000-Hz tone bursts and clicks, found that AP waveforms are not consistently abnormal in acoustic tumours. Abnormally broad APs can be found at all stimulus intensities, or at low intensities only. On the other hand, normal AP waveforms can be recorded at all intensities. Eggermont and his associates tested 33 ears and found that in 23 the AP waveform was consistent with the audiogram. Only 30% showed an abnormally broad AP when related to the audiometric contour.

For derived (frequency-specific) APs, three different unit shapes can be obtained, including the normal biphasic shape; a W-shaped N1, N2 type, found predominantly in Ménière's disease; and a monophasic type observed only in VIIIth nerve tumours or other pontine angle tumours (Eggermont et al 1980). The mere presence of such a monophasic response is a promising detection criterion, but since it is not present in the majority of tumour cases, its general diagnostic value is limited.

Amplitude and Intensity–Amplitude function

The steep slope of the intensity–amplitude function has been used as an indication for the presence of recruitment. Also, it has been noted that the higher the AP threshold, the steeper the intensity–amplitude threshold.

A large number of intensity–amplitude curves in cases of acoustic tumours lie completely within the normal range. When AP thresholds exceed 60 dBnHL, steeply rising intensity–amplitude curves are found, but even at very high intensities the normal values of AP amplitude may not be achieved. Eggermont et al (1980) have suggested that the hearing loss produced by a tumour is at the cochlear level and is indistinguishable from recruiting end-organ lesions when recorded on ECochG.

The observation of the ECochG threshold's being lower than the subjective threshold was made by several investigators. This is associated with medially located tumours. In 27% of patients in a study conducted by Morrison et al (1976), the hearing threshold, as measured by click-evoked AP, was 15 dB lower than the subjective hearing threshold, and it was 15 dB lower in 50% of 14 cases of various cerebello-pontine angle tumours in a study by Eggermont & Odenthal (1977). However, with tone-burst stimulation at 2000, 4000, and 8000 Hz, only in a few cases were ECochG thresholds lower than subjective thresholds (Eggermont et al 1980). These findings relate to medially placed tumours, including acoustic tumours, meningiomas, and gliomas pressing on the brain. Also, a few ears had AP thresholds worse than subjective thresholds. The latter fact has been attributed to the loss of synchrony of the firing neurones and degradation of the response. In general, the threshold obtained with ECochG and subjective hearing methods are in close agreement when tested with more frequency-specific tone bursts, and the difference was abnormal in only 8% of cases (Eggermont et al 1980).

Latency and Latency–Intensity function

Many acoustic tumours produce prolonged latencies of the AP, and in about two-thirds of all cases the latency–intensity curves are distributed above the normal values (Eggermont et al 1980). This abnormality also occurs in cases of severe high-frequency hearing loss and in Ménière's disease (Eggermont 1976). More detailed study of the acoustic-tumour responses, by recording narrow-band AP, shows that they are not above the normal range. This suggests that those prolonged latencies of compound AP evoked by broadband click depend on relative contributions of various narrow-band responses; when hearing loss is mainly in high frequencies, as in acoustic tumours, the contribution is from the lower frequencies, causing prolongation of the latencies.

6. The auditory brainstem response (ABR)

INTRODUCTION

The auditory brainstem response (ABR) represents the far-field potentials recorded from the scalp, and comprises five or more waves generated from the auditory pathway up to the level of the inferior colliculus. The ABR occurs within 10 ms of a click or a brief tone-burst stimulus (see Fig. 6.1). It was originally described by Sohmer & Feinmesser (1967) and independently by Jewett & Williston (1971). As an audiological and a diagnostic test, ABR is firmly established in clinical practice. Its value is most evident in audiometric threshold estimation and in neuro-otological and neurological diagnosis.

GENERATORS OF THE ABR

The extensive literature on the origins of ABR in laboratory animals and in man has been thoroughly reviewed by Buchwald (1983). The early interpretations of the likely origins of ABR have been gained from experimental lesions in animals (Buchwald & Huang 1975), and from human brain structures during operations and in pathological conditions (Moller & Jannetta 1985).

Determining the origins of ABR in laboratory animals and then extrapolating the data to interpret human ABR is not easy. The cochlear nerve is much longer in man than in small mammals (Lang 1981), the volumes of the nuclei differ – for example, the superior olivary complex is smaller in primates than in other mammals (Moore & Moore 1971) – and, in general, the organization of the human auditory system differs in quality from that of the small mammal.

However, the ABR morphology and responsiveness to various experimental manipulations in experimental animals are similar to those in man (Huang & Buchwald 1978, Stockard et al 1978, Don et al 1977).

Apart from peak I, which in both small mammals and man is generated from the distal part of the peripheral nerve, the subsequent peaks are generated from different anatomical structures according to species. For

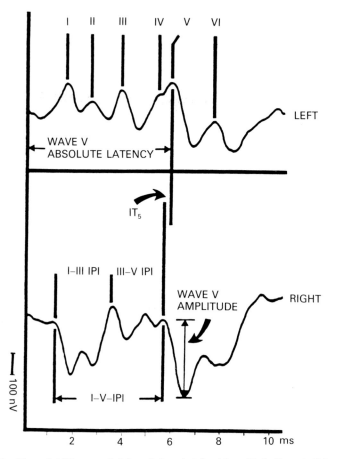

Fig. 6.1 Normal ABRs recorded from left and right sides with ipsilateral click stimulation. The peaks and main diagnostic parameters are shown.

example, wave IV in the cat appears to be analogous to wave V in man (Allen & Starr 1978, Huang 1980).

In man, wave I originates in the distal part of the cochlear nerve, and radiates as a surface negative wave to periauricular sites (Buchwald 1983). The peak latencies of wave I recorded from a surface electrode and from a needle electrode on the promontory have similar values and reflect the gross neural activity of the cochlear nerve (Sohmer & Feinmesser 1967, Abramovich & Billings 1981).

It was thought that wave II originates mainly in the cochlear nucleus (Buchwald 1983). However, intracranial recordings in man suggest that the peak of wave II originates mainly from the proximal part of the cochlear nerve, but with some contributions from the cochlear nucleus (Hashimoto et al 1981, Moller & Jannetta 1985).

The origins of the subsequent waves generated in the brainstem are not

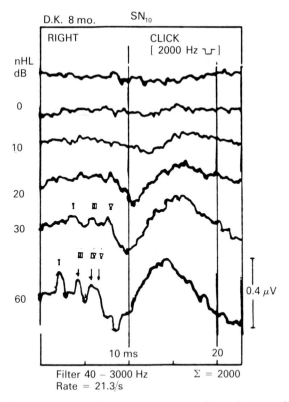

Fig. 6.2 The SN10 response recorded using a band-pass filter of 40–3000 Hz. (After Davis H 1984 with permission.)

clear. It is now accepted that the sequence of the waves does not correspond to simple rostral propagation of the excitation. Most likely, the various orientations of vectorial fields generated in several nuclei overlap, and the studies in man using intracranial recordings support this (Hashimoto et al 1981, Moller & Jannetta 1983, 1985). Peaks III, IV, V, and the subsequent VI and VII derive contributions from more than one anatomical location. Also, each nucleus may contribute to more than one wave in the ABR. Topographic analysis of the auditory-evoked potentials using multichannel recordings, combined with theoretic dipole modelling, suggests that wave III is mainly generated in the region ranging from the ipsilateral cochlear nuclei to the contralateral superior olivary complex, and that the IV–V complex seems to originate from the ipsilateral and contralateral lemniscal structures (Scherg & von Cramon 1985).

One of the most constant morphologic features of the ABR is a vertex–positive peak V, which is followed by a prominent negative potential at the vertex with a latency of 7 ms. This has been named far-field potential 7 (FFP7) by Terkildsen et al (1974). A similar response, especially to low-frequency tone bursts, following wave V at 10 ms is the slow, negative SN10 response shown in Figure 6.2 (Davis & Hirsh 1979). The SN10 is consistent during muscle paralysis, confirming its neural origin (Fria et al 1984).

Each region of the cochlea initiates an ABR from the ascending pathways. Thus, for a click stimulus which excites all of the cochlea, the response that is recorded from a surface electrode is the sum of the responses from all the regions in the cochlea. Each of these 'elemental' responses exhibits the 'travelling wave' delay before its initiation. Thus, the overall ABR is a compound response that represents the sum of the elemental responses. Because of the delays involved, some peaks of the elemental responses are cancelled and some are superimposed. Techniques such as the 'derived-response' method can extract frequency-specific responses from the compound ABR (see p. 37).

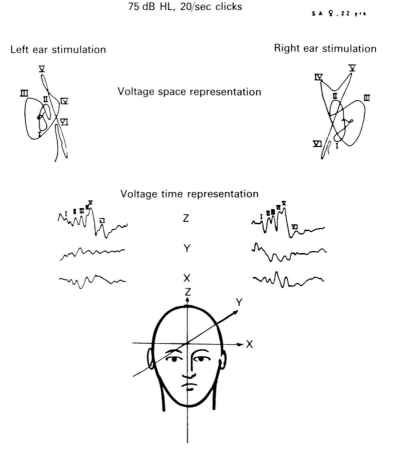

Fig. 6.3 The lower three traces are ABRs, from which the voltage-time and voltage-space representations were derived (top). (After Pratt H et al 1984 with permission.)

Williston et al (1981) and Pratt et al (1984), using three orthogonal electrode pairs, have recorded ABR waveforms and produced three-dimensional representations in voltage-time and voltage-space. When this was done, certain segments of the plot lay in a single plane (Fig. 6.3). Furthermore, the orientation of the plane can be altered by disorders of the auditory system. Current research is refining the interpretation of the data and investigating the effects of various pathologies.

METHODS

Testing environment

The testing environment should exclude extraneous sounds and, in order to minimize muscle activity, provide an environment in which the patient can relax comfortably. The patient is tested in a recumbent position on a couch, as shown in Figure 6.4. A small dose of a muscle relaxant such as diazepam

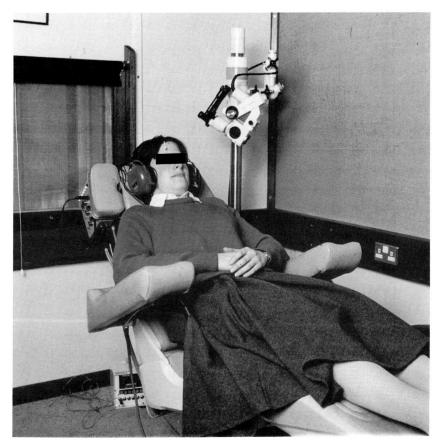

Fig. 6.4 Patient relaxed in the couch prior to ABR recording.

can reduce excessive muscular activity and improve ABR recording in an anxious patient.

A parent or a nurse can make a child patient more relaxed, and, if necessary, sedation or light general anaesthesia can be used in the case of a difficult-to-test child. In neonates, testing after a feed usually insures good test conditions, as the baby often sleeps.

Testing in ideal audiometric conditions in an electrically and acoustically screened audiometric booth is desirable, particularly when the ABR is used for threshold estimation.

Electrode placement

The most commonly used electrode derivation is an active pair connected between mastoid (M) or ear lobe (A) and vertex (Cz). Normative data for ipsilateral mastoid-to-vertex electrode placements are readily available. The earth electrode is placed on the forehead (Fz). To enable bilateral recording in neurological diagnosis, and to minimize the test time when evaluating both ears, one can attach four electrodes at M1, M2, Cz, and Fz to allow M1–Cz and M2–Cz active pairs.

In neonates, the vertex electrode may be moved back towards the occiput, in order to avoid the posterior fontanelle.

There is no general agreement about the waveform polarity, and the results should be given in an unambiguous way. For example, for a mastoid–vertex electrode pair, the ABR peaks (I–V) may be plotted as positive events (vertex-positivity plotted upwards) or as negative events (mastoid-positivity plotted upwards). An example is shown in Figure 6.5.

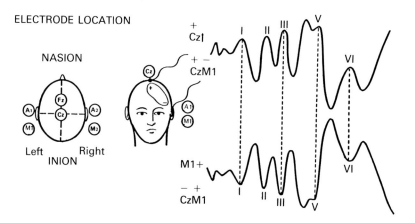

Fig. 6.5 ABR waveforms obtained with a vertex-mastoid electrode pair. The upper trace is obtained when the vertex positivity is plotted upwards. The lower trace is the same waveform with the mastoid positivity plotted upwards.

Technical aspects of stimulation and ABR recording

At present, there is no international standard on stimulation parameters and acquisition of the ABR. However, each laboratory should acquire normative data for specific stimuli, using as guidelines the technical and procedural recommendations of the Electric-Response Audiometry Study Group on ABR measurement (Thornton 1983).

Instrumentation should permit stimulation, both with clicks and tone pips. Monaural stimulation is more commonly used, but binaural stimulation has been suggested for some clinical strategies.

Clicks are generated as electrical pulses of 100 μs duration and are presented through an electrodynamic transducer, such as the Telephonics TDH 39 or TDH 49. Alternating polarity and monophasic stimuli are employed.

Normative data used to provide a baseline for neuro-otological diagnosis are usually acquired at a stimulus-repetition rate of about 10/s at appropriate levels. Reference data obtained at levels from 60 to 100 dBnHL generally provide an adequate baseline. For some neurological applications, an analysis of the ABR recorded from the side contralateral to the one stimulated can help in resolving the diagnosis. Thus, simultaneous bilateral recording can be carried out routinely, as it takes no more test time, but the contralateral data need be analysed only for the few problem cases. For threshold estimation, a higher repetition rate is generally used in order to minimize the test time.

The filter settings, especially for low frequencies, vary according to the application for the ABR (see Ch. 6). For neuro-otologic purposes, the optimal filter settings are 100–3000 Hz.

Normally, at least 1024 sweeps are recommended for a trial average, and the trials are replicated at least once.

NORMATIVE CHARACTERISTIC OF ABR

The criteria for ABR interpretation are based on the waveform morphology, the latencies and the amplitudes of the peaks.

Factors such as age and hearing loss, as well as different stimulus parameters and recording characteristics, can affect the ABR, and these factors are reflected in the inter-laboratory differences in normal data (Thornton 1987).

Waveform of ABR

Assessment of the normal appearance of ABR requires some experience, as it is a subjective, qualitative assessment.

There is considerable variation of the waveform in normal subjects, and, therefore, waveform variation is not a very reliable single feature for clinical evaluation, although some lesions have distinctive response changes. Normally, at high-stimulus intensities, waves I, III, and V can be recognized without difficulty. Wave V is the most prominent wave. Usually, waves IV and V are merged to give a IV/V complex. The peak of wave V is usually more prominent than IV in the complex; however, sometimes the reverse occurs. Waves IV and V may have a clear bifurcation, although sometimes they are completely fused into a broad wave, creating some difficulty in measuring their latencies. At high intensities, a complete bifurcation of wave

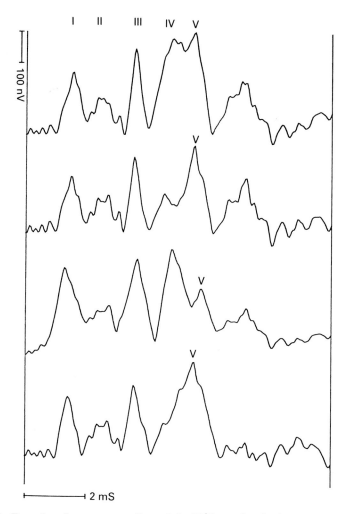

Fig. 6.6 Examples of common recordings of the IV/V complex. In the top trace, IV/V are split, with similar absolute amplitudes. In the trace below, wave IV appears on the rising portion of wave V, in contrast to the next trace in which V appears on the descending portion of wave IV. The lowest trace shows IV as a small inflection on a rising edge of wave V.

I, and sometimes wave III too, can also occur. Examples of normative ABR variations are shown in Figure 6.6.

The contralaterally recorded response has a morphology similar to that described above except that wave I is missing.

ABR latencies

At moderate intensity levels, ABR waves are generally reliable and stable. As a guideline, wave I occurs at about 1.6 ms, and subsequent waves occur approximately at 1-ms intervals. Typical normative ABR latency data are shown in Table 6.1. When the peak of the wave is not defined, the measurement is taken at the beginning of the down slope. The measurement of absolute latency is especially relevant for wave V, which is the most prominent and stable under various conditions, and is, therefore, an important diagnostic parameter.

Inter-peak intervals (IPI) reflect neural transmission and can be affected by lesions of the peripheral nerve and by lesions extrinsic or intrinsic to the brainstem. Clinically, the IPI are measured between the main waves I, III, and V (see Table 6.1). The I–III and III–V IPI are about 2 ms each, and the I–V IPI is approximately 4 ms, and is relatively insensitive to stimulus intensity changes from moderate to high levels (Abramovich & Billings 1981).

The interaural peak difference of wave V (IT 5) is another useful parameter and normally should not exceed 0.3 ms (Fig. 6.1).

ABR amplitude

The peak-to-peak amplitude of the wave components is a less stable parameter than is the peak latency, and it is, therefore, prone to considerable variation in absolute values (see Table 6.1). However, particularly for CNS lesions and for stimulation at fixed levels relative to the individual patient's threshold, the amplitude can give useful diagnostic information (Thornton & Hawkes 1976).

Studies of waveform amplitude variations were carried out by Starr & Achor 1975, Rowe 1978, and Chiappa et al 1979. They found the V/I amplitude ratio to be a valuable clinical parameter. In normal subjects, the V/I ratio is more than 1 and can approximate 3 (Stockard et al 1978).

An example of a diagnostic baseline which uses both amplitude and latency values is shown in Figure 7.17.

Amplitude–intensity and latency–intensity functions

The decreasing intensity of a click stimulus from high levels to threshold alters the waveform, latency, and amplitude of the ABR. Wave V is easily

Table 6.1   Latencies of ABR. Clinical norms. All limits are 95% confidence limits based on data from 17 normal ears. Alternating clicks used. Recording bandwidth 100 Hz–3 kHz.

Latency (ms)

		Click Stimulus Intensity (dBnHL)					
		40	50	60	70	80	90
JI	min.	1.977	1.368	1.281	1.232	1.118	1.021
	mean	2.500	1.863	1.646	1.461	1.311	1.226
	max.	3.022	2.358	2.041	1.690	1.504	1.431
JII	min.	2.453	1.953	2.276	2.188	2.078	2.005
	mean	3.448	2.900	2.738	2.599	2.480	2.361
	max	4.422	3.846	3.199	3.010	2.882	2.717
JIII	min.	3.908	3.391	3.145	3.254	3.086	3.033
	mean	4.514	4.037	3.706	3.564	3.426	3.387
	max.	5.120	4.683	4.267	3.874	3.766	3.741
JIV	min.	4.087	4.114	4.181	4.234	4.164	4.176
	mean	5.564	5.179	4.919	4.779	4.678	4.622
	max.	7.040	6.243	5.656	5.324	5.191	5.067
JV	min.	5.446	5.315	5.034	5.113	4.981	4.958
	mean	6.371	6.044	5.656	5.498	5.425	5.329
	max.	7.295	6.772	6.277	5.883	5.868	5.699
JVI	min.	7.186	6.778	6.454	6.404	6.310	6.269
	mean	8.025	7.683	7.363	7.111	6.971	6.959
	max.	8.864	8.587	8.271	7.818	7.631	7.648

Inter-aural peak differences (L–R)

		Stimulus Amplitude (dBnHL)					
		40	50	60	70	80	90
IT5	min.	−1.083	−0.636	−0.551	−0.376	−0.368	−0.311
	mean	−0.041	0.164	−0.192	0.017	−0.074	−0.099
	max.	1.001	0.963	0.168	0.409	0.221	0.114

Inter-peak intervals

		Stimulus Amplitude (dBnHL)					
		40	50	60	70	80	90
JIII-JI	min.	1.761	1.633	1.604	1.097	1.795	1.718
	mean	2.027	2.162	2.046	2.103	2.115	2.161
	max.	2.292	2.690	2.487	2.299	2.435	2.603
JV-JI	min.	2.912	3.806	3.535	3.730	3.599	3.684
	mean	3.873	4.155	3.995	4.037	4.114	4.103
	max.	4.833	4.504	4.454	4.344	4.629	4.521
JV-JIII	min.	1.063	1.416	1.441	1.629	1.539	1.561
	mean	1.855	2.007	1.949	1.934	1.999	1.942
	max.	2.646	2.598	2.457	2.239	2.459	2.322

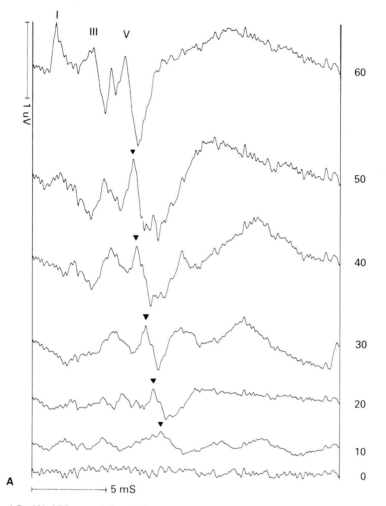

Fig. 6.7 (**A**) ABR recorded at different intensities from an adult patient. (**B**) The corresponding amplitude and latency I/O function.

recognizable in normal subjects and is identifiable down to 20 dBnHL, whereas the earlier waves become difficult to identify below 50 dBnHL (Fig. 6.7). At 20-dBnHL click stimulus, the amplitude of wave V is about 0.3 μV, compared to 0.6 μV at 70 dBnHL (Picton et al 1981). Threshold estimation is based on detection of wave V, which, for normal subjects can be visualized in 75% of cases at 10–20 dBnHL and can be seen in all cases at higher sound levels. Wave III is identifiable in about 60% of subjects at 30 dBnHL, and wave I in 75% at 50 dBnHL (Worthington & Peters 1980).

A decrease in intensity will prolong all wave latencies. The latency of wave V is about 5.9 ms at 70 dBnHL and increases to about 7.7 ms at

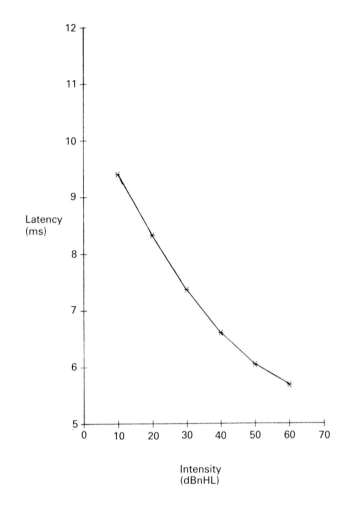

B

Intensity
(dBnHL)

20 dBnHL, thus giving an average shift in wave V slope of 30–40 μs per dBnHL (Picton et al 1981, Schwartz & Berry 1985). However, the latency–intensity function slope is non-linear (Fig. 6.8).

SUBJECT CHARACTERISTICS OF THE NORMAL ABR

The ABR in neonates and in the developing child

The morphology, amplitude, and latency of ABR are age-dependent in the developing auditory system, a dependency mainly attributed to myelination and synaptic efficiency (Shah et al 1978), as well as to the growing skull (Jacobson et al 1981).

Clear ABR responses can be recorded as early as 28 weeks in premature infants (Starr et al 1977). By the gestational age of 40 weeks, one can trace

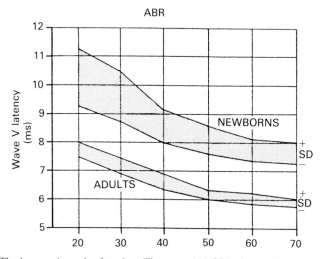

Fig. 6.8 The latency–intensity function. The mean (±1 SD) of wave V latencies obtained from normal neonates (top) and adults (bottom). (Reproduced with permission from Shallop J K et al 1984.)

ABR threshold to clicks of 30 dBnHL or lower. However, in neonates and infants, ABR responses differ from those of adults.

Waveform

The waveform morphology of an infant's response at relatively high intensity clicks (70 dBnHL) is easily identified, usually consisting of three prominent waves, as shown in Figure 6.9. These waves correspond to adult waves I, III, and V. Waves II and IV are often not seen, but by the age of 1 year, all five waves can be identified. Wave I appears between the 27th and 30th week of conceptual age, and wave V at about 32 weeks (Stockard et al 1983).

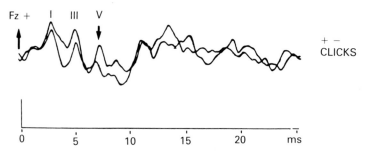

Fig. 6.9 ABR recorded in a neonate. Waves I, III, and V are well defined, but have longer latencies than do adult values.

Amplitude

The amplitudes are smallest in neonates. During the first 3 months of age, the amplitude of wave I increases and may become twice the size of that recorded from an adult. This can be explained by the electrode's location on the undeveloped mastoid being nearer to the cochlear nerve than in an adult, because of the smaller head size (Salamy et al 1979). Wave V in a neonate has a smaller amplitude than in an adult, but reaches the adult values by the age of 12 months. Wave III has a similar pattern of development (Hecox & Burkhard 1982).

As in adults, the absolute amplitudes in neonates and infants are prone to considerable variations; however, the relative ratio of V/I can be used as a clinical parameter. The amplitude ratio V/I is about 1, which is smaller than in adults (Hecox et al 1981). However, the adult values are reached soon after 1 year of age (Salamy et al 1982).

Latency

The absolute latencies of all ABR components in neonates are prolonged. During the maturation period, wave I reaches adult values by 3 months of age, and wave V after 1–2 years of age. Wave III follows the maturation pattern of wave V (Salamy & McKean 1976, Jacobson et al 1982, Salamy et al 1982). The normative data for click stimuli from some investigators are presented in Figure 6.10.

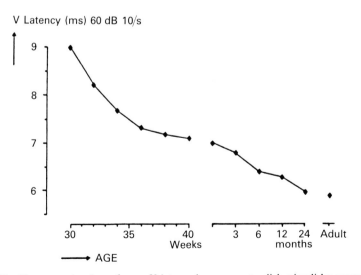

Fig. 6.10   The normative data of wave V latency in response to click stimuli by gestational age. (Reproduced with permission of Picton T W et al 1981.)

The inter-peak latencies are also prolonged. At term, the IPI for waves I–V is about 5 ms, and within 1–2 years the adult value of 4 ms is reached. However, clinically, the latency–age function is prone to variation and is not precise enough to assess the infant's gestational age to within 2 weeks. Furthermore, the agreement is poor with the age estimated by the mother's last menstrual period (Galambos & Despland 1980). In the developing infant's auditory pathway, the latencies of the ABR change in the same way as stimulus intensity in adults, and the inter-peak latencies IPI I–V, I–III, and III–V are practically intensity-independent.

Effect of ageing on ABR

It is thought that ageing can also influence ABR. Rowe's (1978) data showed that wave-V latency increased by 0.3–0.5 ms for subjects aged 51–74 years as compared to subjects aged 17–33 years. Jerger & Hall (1980) showed a 0.2-ms latency increase in normal subjects aged 20–59 years. Maurizi et al (1982) compared young subjects and subjects with a mean age of 62 years with hearing levels on the audiogram of better than 30 dB, and found that the latency of wave V was prolonged by 0.2 ms in the older group. However, some investigators did not find a significant latency increase in young normal subjects and in subjects over 60 years of age (Beagley & Sheldrake 1978, Rosenhamer et al 1980).

In general, it is thought that in patients over 50 years of age with reasonably good hearing, the effect of age should be taken into consideration (Fig. 6.11).

Gender

The latency of wave V and the IPI for waves I–V are significantly longer in males than in females of the same age (Beagley & Sheldrake 1978, Stockard et al 1978, Jerger & Hall 1980, Rosenhamer et al 1980). According to Schwartz & Berry (1985), the wave-V latency for males is 0.14 ms longer, on average, than for females. They also found that the amplitudes of the waves are slightly greater in females than in males. An accepted explanation for such slight differences in adults is that female heads are smaller, and the auditory pathway between the cochlear nerve and the midbrain shorter.

In neonates, the latency differences between the sexes are not observed.

Body temperature

The circadian variation and decrease in body temperature by 1°C have been found to prolong the latency of wave V by 0.2 ms (Marshall & Douchin 1981, Picton et al 1981).

Temperatures below 35°C prolong the latency of wave V by 0.25 ms/1°C temperature drop (Stockard et al 1978). This results in a corresponding prolongation of IPI in waves I–V; for example, a core temperature of 32°C

Wave V latency (ms)

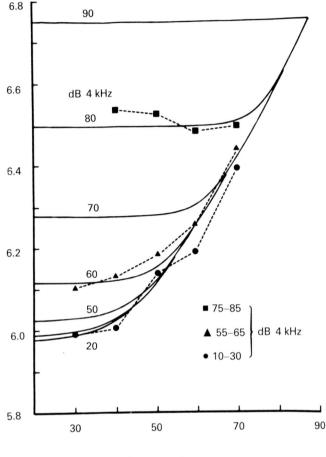

Fig. 6.11 Data and a fitted model of mean wave-V latency to show effects of age (Abramovich S J & Hyde M, unpublished.)

leads to an increase in I–V intervals of about 0.75 ms. This effect is related to hypothermia and should be noted when monitoring the neurological status of a comatose patient or during per-operative monitoring of ABR. Similar findings are obtained in hypothyroidism in which the patient's body temperature is below normal (Thornton & Ghariani 1990).

Sedatives and anaesthetic agents

Volatile anaesthetics like nitrous oxide and halothane do not seem to have a significant effect on human ABR during general anaesthesia, according to

Stockard et al (1980). Similarly, no effect on the latencies was reported with clinical doses of pethidine, diazepam, and barbiturates, although the amplitudes of later peaks were slightly reduced. The ABR is also unaltered by the neuromuscular blocking agents used in preparation for intubation (Kileny & McIntyre 1985). However, relatively minor dose-related effects on the III–V interval have been reported as a result of the use of enflurane and halothane in nitrous oxide (Fig. 6.12) (Thornton et al 1984, Jones et al 1985). The III–V interval was significantly increased with halothane concentrations of about 1.5%. Intravenous anaesthetic agents such as etomidate and althesin had no effect on the ABR (Jones et al 1985).

However, pharmacological agents such as lignocaine, used systemically, may cause changes in ABR morphology (Jave et al 1982), and acute ethanol intoxication has been reported to cause prolongation of IPI in waves I–V (Rosenhamer 1981). Alterations of ABR have also been noted in comatose patients as barbiturates levels increased (Schwartz & Berry 1985).

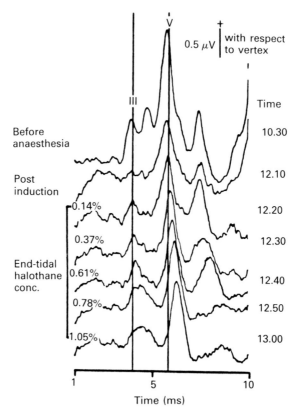

Fig. 6.12 The effect of anaesthesia on the ABR. Note relatively minor dose-related increase of latencies III and V. (Reproduced with permission from Thornton C et al 1984.)

INSTRUMENTATION FACTORS INFLUENCING NORMAL ABR

Several methodological factors may influence the ABR. These include band-pass filtering, artefact rejection, common-mode rejection, and electrode impedance. These factors have been discussed in Chapter 3. Stimulus phase and repetition rate also alter the ABR.

Filter characteristics

The spectral components of the ABR waveform range from about 50 to a little over 1000 Hz (Kevanishvili & Aponchenko 1979, Laukli & Mair 1981). However, the filtering that provides maximum waveform fidelity is not what is required in the clinic. The filter settings vary according to the application for the ABR.

If wave V is to be used to estimate threshold, then maximum detectability of wave V is required, and waveform distortion does not matter as long as wave-V amplitude is maximized. There is a low-frequency component of the brainstem response which enhances wave V at the cost of decreasing the amplitudes of adjacent peaks. Thornton (1984) has reported the results of a digital filtering experiment which showed that wave-V amplitude is maximized for low-frequency limits of 20–40 Hz for the filter slopes most commonly encountered.

If the ABR is to be used for neurological or neuro-otological diagnosis, then all of the peaks are important, and the compromise frequency best for maximizing all responses is approximately 100 Hz for the low-frequency limit.

The high-frequency limit remains the same for all applications; it is generally around 2000–3000 Hz.

It is important to realize that analogue filters produce propagation delays, and these delays increase as the bandwidth gets narrower. When calculating latencies, one must allow for the propagation delay of the recording filter so that no errors are introduced; Thornton (1984) comments on this. A possible but, at the moment, expensive solution would be to use digital filters, which can have zero phase shifts, in order to overcome the problems inherent in analogue filters (Boston & Ainslie 1980).

Stimulus polarity

In recording the neurogenic response, alternating polarity stimuli have been advocated because polarity-sensitive components such as artefacts and the CM will be cancelled (Salt & Thornton 1984). Subjectively, click stimuli of opposite phase are indistinguishable, and do not seem to offer conclusive evidence of significant spectral differences between the rarefaction and condensation clicks (Picton et al 1981, Maurer et al 1980).

The polarity-dependent amplitude and morphology of ABR waves have been described in many studies; however contradictory conclusions have been reported (Pijl 1987).

Wave-I latency decreases by 0.04–0.07 ms, and its amplitude usually increases significantly when rarefaction, as compared to condensation stimuli are used (Stockard et al 1979, Coats & Martin 1977, Picton et al 1981, Kevanishvili & Aponchenko 1981, Ruth et al 1982). This is possibly due to the fact that the rarefaction click initiates the basilar membrane's movement towards the scala vestibuli, and when one records the peak firing rate of a neural fibre on the histogram, the response appears earlier in relation to rarefaction stimulus as compared with condensation stimulus, although the envelopes of the histograms are similar (Antoli-Candela & Kiang 1978). However, it has been reported that in 17% of normal subjects, wave I is shorter in response to condensation clicks, while 22% of the population do not show any difference (Stockard et al 1980).

Latency shifts of wave I are not necessarily transmitted to subsequent wave peaks (Pijl 1987). Generally, it is thought that waves III and V show no consistent latency differences in recorded responses to both rarefaction and condensation clicks (Terkildsen et al 1973, Borg & Lofqvist 1982, Kevanishvili & Aponchenko 1981). The explanation for this could be that components III and V are generated in relation to the discharge envelope pattern of the auditory fibre, rather than in relation to initial onset of the discharge (Picton et al 1981).

The mean IPI I–V values have been reported to be longer for rarefaction than for condensation clicks by 0.07 ms in adults, and by 0.03 ms in neonates; this effect is even greater at the rapid-click presentation rate (Stockard et al 1979). However, Pijl (1987) has reported large polarity-related IPI I–V shifts between rarefaction and condensation (R–C) clicks in individual cases, ranging from +0.28 to −0.42 ms in a normal hearing group.

Rarefaction stimuli are more effective than condensation stimuli in eliciting a complete sequence of identifiable waves, especially peaks I through IV (Stockard & Stockard 1983, Sand & Sulg 1984, Pijl 1987). Inversion of stimulus phase has been recommended as a strategy for separating the fused IV/V complex when the wave-V latency measurement is problematic (Maurer 1985).

Salt & Thornton (1984) have shown that, even among normal subjects, some individuals give a much better response to condensation stimuli, whilst others give a much better response to rarefaction stimuli. They recommend that, for clinical purposes, the responses to both polarities should be recorded separately. If these responses do not differ, they can be averaged to give a final waveform. If one is much better than the other, diagnostic decisions should be based on the better waveform.

For practical purposes, the latencies of waves I to V are relatively stable, with inversion of the stimulus phase in normal hearing or mild degrees of hearing loss. However, the proportion of I–V intervals, that changed their values by more than 0.2 ms when the stimulus polarity was changed, is increased for high frequency hearing losses of more than 40 dB (Pijl 1987). Because of this, summation of slightly out-of-phase shifted peaks of ABR obtained with clicks of opposite acoustic phase may result partly in response degradation.

Repetition-rate function

In general, an increased latency and decreased amplitude of the ABR components have been found to accompany increase of stimulation rate (Pratt & Sohmer 1976).

For neuro-otologic purposes, the rate of stimulation should not be more than 12/s; otherwise, the resultant adaptation may compromise the clarity of early waves I and III, and hence the estimation of the inter-peak intervals. However, it has been suggested that by exerting stress on the auditory system with high-repetition-rate stimuli, it may be possible to detect incipient abnormalities in the brainstem (Robinson & Rudge 1977).

The wave-V amplitude is not markedly affected until the stimulus rate exceeds 30/s (Hyde et al 1976). It is acceptable to use higher rates in order to save time when assessing the hearing threshold. A further increase in stimulation rate has more considerable effect on both the latencies and the amplitudes.

If the stimulus-presentation rate is increased from 10 to 80/s, the amplitudes of waves I and III decrease to 50% of their initial values; however, wave V is more stable, and its amplitude decreases to 90% of its initial value (Picton et al 1981).

As regards the latencies, Picton et al (1981) found that using 70 dBnHL clicks of alternating polarity and increasing the rate of stimulation from 10 to 80/s, caused an increase of the latencies of waves I, III, and V by 0.14, 0.23, and 0.39 ms, respectively. The normative rate criteria were suggested by Musiek & Collegly (1985), who allowed a 0.1 ms shift of latency in wave V for every 10 clicks/s increase in rate. For example, a rate increase from 10 to 50 clicks/s is expected to increase wave V latency by 0.4 ms.

The IPI of waves I–V also increases correspondingly with the stimulation rate. On the other hand, wave I latency shifts are more affected by polarity and intensity of the stimulus than are those of wave V. Therefore, the rate-related IPI are more difficult to predict (Stockard & Stockard 1983). The effect of increased repetition rate on the IPI of waves I–V seems to be less for condensation than for rarefaction clicks (Stockard et al 1979).

Relatively small latency changes for wave I with increasing click stimulation rate could be due to a more rapid adaptation of the higher frequencies of the auditory fibres. Therefore, the main cochlear origin of the response is slightly shifted more apically along the basilar membrane, and the latency of wave I increases a little (Eggermont 1976, Charlet de Sauvage & Aran 1976, Mouney et al 1978).

Greater increase in the latencies of the later components in response to increasing stimulus-repetition rate could be explained by central synaptic adaptation, and/or by a different population of cochlear fibres contributing to different components of the response (Picton et al 1981).

The effects of high-repetition rates depend upon the maturity of the auditory pathway. With increasing repetition rates, the difference between a full-term neonate and an adult, for all waves and IPI, increases; this has been attributed to the underdevelopment of the auditory pathway (Morgan et al 1987).

Number of samples

In threshold estimation, as the stimulus intensity is decreased, the number of sweeps should be increased in order to improve signal-to-noise ratio and give an adequate resolution of wave V. Usually, two superimposed ABR recordings at threshold, each composed of at least 2000 averages, will give satisfactory responses.

Effect of masking

Interaural attenuation for click stimuli has been estimated to be about 50 dB (Reid & Thornton 1983). The ipsilaterally recorded brainstem responses to stimuli presented to right and left ears are largely independent. Also, any effect of binaural interaction is relatively small and is decreased by low levels of masking (Picton et al 1981). Broad-band noise masking is an effective audiological method to exclude participation of the non-tested ear, and, according to Reid & Thornton (1983), contralateral masking has only a minimal effect on the ABR.

Transducer types

The unwanted post-stimulus oscillations of the transducer, or 'ringing effect', can interact with the stimulus. Also, the electromagnetic artefacts of electrodynamic earphones can affect the early components of ABR. However, the latter artefacts can be avoided by shielding the earphones. The difference in acoustic spectrum between clicks transduced through different earphones, or between shielded and unshielded earphones, may be significant, and this can reflect on ABR morphology and latencies, particularly at lower intensities. Different ear cushions have different couplings with the external ear, and even this can introduce some alterations in the response (Coats & Kidder 1980). Therefore, it is important to specify the spectral characteristics of the earphone.

The stimuli delivered from the loudspeaker at a distance of 0.5 m from the ear will introduce a delay of about 1.7 ms.

The bone conductors also introduce time delay. The bone conductors have acoustic energy spectra usually limited to 2500 Hz, and, therefore, the transduced click excites the basilar membrane more apically compared to a click stimulus transduced by earphones with a wider spectrum. This leads to about a 0.5-ms latency shift of the ABR response at the same level of acoustic output.

AUDIOMETRIC FREQUENCY SPECIFICITY OF THE ABR

In this section, various aspects of frequency specificity will be considered. Firstly, we consider the use of various masking techniques applied to click stimuli; then tone-pip stimulation and tone pip in masking noise.

Threshold responses with clicks

The ABR reflects electrical epiphenomena along the auditory pathway up to the level of the inferior colliculus. However, ABR can be correlated with behavioural thresholds, and, therefore, can be used for the interpretation of hearing in a population that cannot be satisfactorily tested by behavioural audiometry. The ABR can be recorded non-invasively, and it is little affected by sleep, sedation, or general anaesthesia.

Auditory-threshold measurement is based on the most prominent wave, wave V, since it can be detected to within 15 dB of the behavioural threshold (Kaga & Tanaka 1980). Thus, if the stimulus generator can produce clicks up to 100 dBnHL, then wave V can be used to measure thresholds up to 80–85 dB. No recordable response implies a threshold greater than this. In normal adults, wave I is not present on the recording, if the click intensity is lower than about 50 dB above the subjective hearing level.

The click thresholds do not reflect hearing loss at lower frequencies, for example, 500 Hz, nor, sometimes, at very high frequencies such as 4000 Hz and above. Several investigators have reported that normal thresholds for broad-spectrum click-evoked ABR can be recorded when pure-tone audiograms show significant losses at a single frequency between 500 and 6000 Hz (Picton et al 1979, Yamada et al 1979).

Thus, the use of clicks in relation to ABR may not reflect precise, frequency-specific audiometric contour and, in general, the ABR threshold, for losses that are approximately flat, correlates best with audiometric thresholds of 2–3 kHz.

Frequency-specific responses using masked clicks

In order to improve the frequency-specificity of click-evoked ABR, a number of techniques have been tried. Using a broad-band click, one can restrict the responsive cochlear region to a specific place on the basilar membrane, while using masking noise in the same ear (Smith 1979, Geisler & Sinex

1980, Pickles 1982). However, it is known that masking of low frequencies tends to spread the masking effect to regions of higher frequencies, and so high-pass masking (see p. 37) is a safer method.

Those frequency-specific ABR responses relaying on ipsilateral simultaneous masking methods include: clicks in band-reject noise (notched masking noise), derived-responses obtained by using clicks in high-pass masking noise, and derived-responses obtained by using clicks and narrow-band masking noise or tone (see p. 37).

Clicks in notched noise

ABR responses to clicks in notched noise (see Fig. 3.10) have distinct waves III and V, but the responses are very small, on average 0.18 μV at 70 dBnHL across frequencies. The method is further complicated, because the notch width, level of masking, and band-pass of the filters of the recording amplifiers have different effects on ABR response (Zanten & Brocaar 1984, Stapells et al 1985). The response does not correlate very well with the pure-tone audiometric data, according to Pratt et al (1984), and, therefore, this method is not recommended.

Derived-response using narrow-band masking

Frequency-specific responses can be obtained by using a specific masking tone or a narrow-band noise (Stapells et al 1985) (see p. 37 and Fig. 3.10A). There is also some spread of masking from nominal frequency towards higher frequencies, making this method complicated for clinical use.

Derived-response using clicks in high-pass masking noise

A frequency-specific ABR response can be obtained by simultaneously presenting click and high-pass masking noise to the same ear. A specific portion of the cochlea can be masked. The advantage of high-pass masking, as compared to low- or band-pass masking, is that there is no unwanted spread of masking into the higher frequencies.

By altering the cut-off frequency of the high-pass masking noise and repeating the procedure, a series of high-pass masked responses can be obtained. Paired subtraction of these waveforms produces a set of derived-responses covering several frequencies (Parker & Thornton 1978, Eggermont & Don 1980) (see Fig. 3.11). For example, if a click and high-pass masking noise with a cut-off frequency of 4000 Hz is presented to the ear, then the response (A) will be generated from the unmasked 0–4000 Hz region of the cochlea. Next, the high-pass filter is set, for example, to 3000 Hz, and response (B) will come from a smaller region of the cochlea at 0–3000 Hz. By subtracting response (A) from response (B), a derived-response between the 3000- and 4000-Hz region of the cochlea is obtained.

Recording derived-responses allows audiometric estimation even at low frequencies. High-pass masking cut-offs at 500 Hz still give a clear wave V with a latency that is about 4 ms longer than the latency of an unmasked response. However, data from cat studies have shown the low frequency response to be less reliable than those obtained at high frequencies. As the centre frequency of the derived-response decreases from 4000 to 500 Hz, the latency of wave V increases by approximately 4 ms. The responses generated in the 4000 Hz and 2000 Hz regions in the cochlea show wave components, I, III, and V at high-intensity stimuli. But below the 2000-Hz region, the responses show only broad wave V component (Stapells et al 1985). Normal thresholds for derived-responses are generally within 25 dBnHL at 1000, 2000, and 4000 Hz, but within 30–40 dBnHL at 500 Hz (Stapells et al 1985).

Comparing frequency-specific methods using masking clicks, one may conclude that the derived-response method is probably the best approach.

ABR responses to tone pips

Attempts to improve frequency specificity have been made by using tone pips (Davis 1976). High frequency tone-pip responses approximate the audiogram (Terkildsen et al 1975, Mitchell & Clemis 1977). A problem with low-frequency stimuli below 1000 Hz is that they do not have the sharp onset necessary for good ABR generation, and only wave V is recordable (Fig. 6.13).

The main stimulus parameters for brief tones are frequency, rise-time, and intensity. Decreasing the frequency of the tone from 4000 to 500 Hz

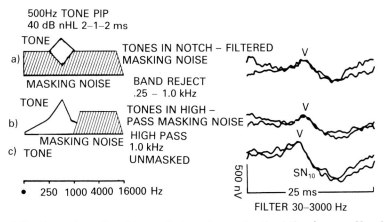

Fig. 6.13 Comparison of masking methods and tone-pip stimulation for wave V and SN10. The top trace shows the waveform for a 500-Hz tone in notched noise. The middle trace is the waveform obtained from the tone in a high-pass filtered masking noise. The bottom trace shows the unmasked response. (Recordings with permission from Hyde M 1985.)

increases the latency of wave V, reflecting the time necessary for the travel-ling wave to reach apical regions in the cochlea. The amplitude of wave V remains nearly constant in response to low and high frequency stimuli, providing that the recording amplifiers have a sufficiently low frequency limit.

The rise-time of the stimulus affects both the latency and the amplitude of the ABR. With increase of the rise-time, the latency of wave V increases and the amplitude decreases (Stapells & Picton 1981). This is particularly relevant for lower tone frequencies. Rise-time increase also leads to less synchronization of neuronal response and to prolongation of the latency of wave V. Increasing the rise-time while keeping the slope constant produces no further change in latency or amplitude after a critical duration is reached; this duration is about 2 ms for a 2000 Hz stimulus (Kodera et al 1983). It is thought that at this point most of the fibres involved in generation of ABR response are activated (Brinkman & Scherg 1979).

Threshold estimation based on detection of wave V is more difficult at lower frequencies for purely technical reasons. Providing that appropriate recording bandwidths are used for stimuli below 1000 Hz, wave V can be detected with some certainty to within 20 dB of the threshold. Several in-vestigators (Suzuki & Horiuchi 1977, Stapells & Picton 1981) have sug-gested lowering the high-pass filter setting from the more usual settings to 10 or even 0.5 Hz.

Davis & Hirsh (1979) identified a vertex negative wave appearing as the trough after ABR wave V, and called it 'slow negative wave at 10 ms', or SN10. This wave is enhanced by distortion of the waveform by the pre-amplifier filter (Picton et al 1981, Doyle & Hyde 1981) (Fig. 6.13).

The cochlear sites contributing to ABR generation using tone-pip stimuli may differ substantially from the nominal tone frequency (Picton et al 1979). However, there is evidence that one can restrict the excited cochlear region by simultaneously using masking noise in the same ear as tone-pip stimuli. ABR thresholds obtained in such a way agree well with the audiogram (Stapells & Picton 1981).

Frequency-specific responses using masked tones

Using various masking methods to limit responsiveness of different regions in the cochlea, Burkard & Hecox (1983) demonstrated that the responses to high intensity, low frequency unmasked brief tones originate in the basal turn of the cochlea.

It is known that in subjects with high frequency hearing loss the brief-tone ABR threshold may be incorrectly estimated because of energy spread towards the more sensitive low frequencies. Because of the acoustic characteristics of brief tones and their audiometric contours, frequency-specific ABR responses may not be obtained. However, by using tech-niques of presenting brief tones simultaneously with masking noise in the same ear, one can improve the frequency specificity of ABR by reducing responsiveness in the masked regions of the cochlea.

Tones in high-pass masking noise

By simultaneously presenting tones and high-pass masking noise in the same ear, one can obtain frequency-specific responses (see Fig. 6.13), and this is a valuable method, especially for low frequency tones (Kileny 1981, Laukli 1983). The advantage of high-pass masking is that there is no spread of masking from low frequencies, as occurs, for example, in notched-noise masking. For a 500 Hz tone, Stapells et al (1985) recommend noise intensities of 0, 10, or 20 dB below the dBpeSPL of the tone, and the high-pass noise cut-off at 1300 Hz with a slope of 60 dB/octave.

Tones in notched-noise masking

Tones can be presented in ipsilateral, notch-filtered masking noise, which is a variation of band-reject filtered noise (Fig. 6.14). Wide notches with cut-off points one octave above and below the nominal frequency of brief-tone stimuli and the slope of the notch of 48 dB/octave can be used (Hyde 1985). The intensity of masking noise for tones is lower than the levels required to mask clicks. Also, tones in notched noise provide a greater concentration of stimulus energy in the desired frequency than do clicks in notched noise. Stapells et al (1985) recommend tones with rise, plateau, and fall times of 2, 1, and 2 ms, respectively, in a noise level 20 dB below the dBpeSPL of the tone, and a notch of one octave in width and at least

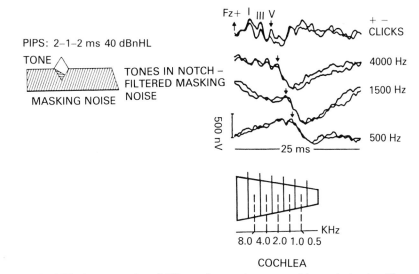

Fig. 6.14 ABRs from tone pips of different frequencies presented in notched noise. (From *Laryngoscope* 1983, 93: 1118, with permission.)

20 dB in depth. For low frequency tone-evoked ABR, the bandwidth of 20–2000 Hz is recommended.

This technique provides good agreement with the pure-tone audiogram (Picton et al 1979) and has been used in estimating hearing in infants (Alberti et al 1983). It is a quicker and probably more efficient method than using derived-responses for audiometric assessment; however, it requires more complicated noise-masking filters.

Conclusion

Click ABR audiometry has valuable accuracy in many cases; however, the absence of frequency-specific information is a definite limitation. ABR audiometry with only brief tones does not guarantee frequency specificity, but is is possible to measure frequency-specific thresholds by simultaneously presenting tone or click stimulus and one of the masking-noise methods in the same ear.

In a relaxed adult or a sleeping infant, frequency-specific ABR gives a threshold sensitivity of about 20 dB for audiometric frequencies above 500 Hz, and of about 30 dB at 500 Hz. This means that at 500 Hz, for hearing losses of 70 dB or more, it is difficult to estimate threshold with ABR. At higher audiometric frequencies, hearing losses of up to 80 dB should be resolved with ABR.

7. The ABR in hearing disorders and auditory dysfunction

ABR IN CONDUCTIVE HEARING LOSS

Evaluation of the type of hearing disorder is of importance, especially in a child. When pure-tone audiometry is not possible, tympanometry is of great assistance. However, it should be pointed out that tympanometry has its limitations when the patient is under 7 months of age (Paradise 1982). Conductive hearing loss can be estimated by ABR, and it is important to recognize this disorder because it may lead to incorrect interpretation of ABR results and may mimic ABR changes due to cochlear and retrocochlear pathologies.

Pathophysiology of the ABR

It is well recognized that conductive hearing loss prolongs the latencies of all ABR waves when air-conduction stimuli are used. This is due to stimulus energy-level reduction (McGee & Clemis 1982), and is equivalent to normative wave-V latency shifts with stimulus-intensity change.

Conductive-loss effect on the latencies of ABR

Prolongation of the latency of wave V by 0.3–0.4 ms for every 10 dB of conductive hearing loss has been estimated by several investigators, and this is similar to the prolongation of latency due to the decrease of stimulus intensity in normal subjects (Fria & Sabo 1980, Finitzo-Hieber & Friel-Patti 1985).

In young infants, the latency of wave I is less age-dependent than is that of wave V, because the latency of wave I matures within the first 6 weeks, but that of wave V matures much later, within 12–18 months. Therefore, for estimation of conductive hearing loss in infants, the prolongation of wave I may be preferred to that of wave V as a parameter.

Correspondingly, the inter-peak latency in IPI I–V is normal in conductive hearing loss. However, in moderate to severe hearing loss, wave I may not be identifiable, and prolongation of the latency of wave V may lead to an incorrect interpretation of the type of hearing dysfunction, if only the

ABR results are considered. Clearly, there are standard methods of determining conductive losses which have to be used in conjunction with ABR.

Latency–intensity function

Estimation of the latency–intensity function may help in resolving the problem of type of hearing loss. The latency–intensity function is displaced proportionally to the amount of conductive hearing loss and is parallel to the normal slope, as shown in Figure 7.1.

Although this function may be consistent with conductive hearing loss, it is not diagnostic. Various pathologies, specifically CNS lesions, can also produce the result of Figure 7.1, but may be distinguished from conductive losses by the value of the I–V interval.

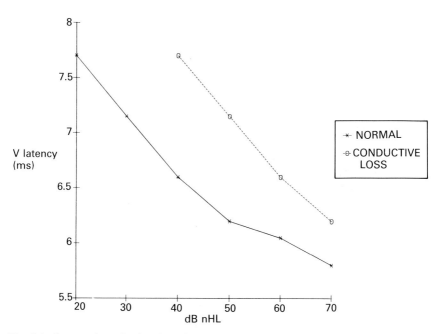

Fig. 7.1 Latency–intensity function of wave V in conductive hearing loss. The function is parallel to the normal slope.

Estimation of conductive hearing loss

Conductive hearing loss can be estimated by plotting the wave V latency–intensity function of the patient and comparing it with normal values. If the stimulus intensity is plotted on the horizontal axis, the amount of conductive loss is equal to the amount that the patient's curve is shifted to the right of the normal values (see Fig. 7.1). For 70% of the subjects studied by Fria & Sabo (1980), the estimated hearing loss was within 5 dB of the subjective audiogram at frequencies 500, 1000, and 2000 Hz, and within 10 dB at 4000 Hz.

Mild middle-ear pathology or serious otitis media with a C-type tympanogram may not prolong the latency of ABR.

Some investigators do not use the latency–intensity function for conductive hearing estimation, because, for a given latency value for wave V, the hearing loss can vary as much as 20 dB (Eggermont 1982). However, estimates taken from several points on an I/O function can improve the accuracy.

Bone-conduction ABR

Impedance measurements should be used to improve conductive hearing loss diagnosis, but when this is not feasible in neonates or infants with external meatal atresia, bone-conduction, click-evoked ABR can be helpful in evaluating cochlear reserve.

Masking of the contralateral ear is as essential in assessing bone conduction as in conventional audiometry.

The responses obtained using a bone conductor are longer by 0.4 ms than air-conducted clicks at the same intensity. This is because bone-conductors limit the spectral energy of the click to lower frequencies. Theoretically, therefore, with bone conductors, the response comes from the lower-frequency region in the cochlea (Finitzo-Hieber & Friel-Patti 1985).

In the absence of both a latency I/O function and I–V interval values, the definite diagnosis of conductive hearing loss and its relative contribution to overall hearing loss can be completely assessed only by doing air- and bone-conduction ABR.

ABR IN COCHLEAR HEARING LOSS

Pathophysiology of ABR

Several pathophysiologic factors due to cochlear lesion may lead to ABR changes. For example, inadequate synchronization and loss of tuning function of the primary neurones associated with cochlear lesions may occur, consequently affecting the ABR.

Severe cochlear hearing loss due to depletion of hair cells at the basal region may result in prolongation of latencies as a result of the longer time for the travelling wave to reach the responding regions on the basilar membrane.

Audiometric contour may also affect the ABR. For example, high-frequency hearing loss may have greater effect on wave I than on wave V, because generators of wave I contribute relatively more from the basal region.

Waveform and amplitude of ABR

Wave V is the most prominent and constant wave on ABR recording in cochlear hearing loss, appearing within 20 dB of sensation level. All five waves usually appear clearly when the click stimulus intensity is more than 50 dB above the hearing level.

In a high frequency hearing loss of more than 50 dBnHL, wave I cannot be identified with confidence in most cases (Fig. 7.2). At some point, hearing loss of cochlear origin eliminates the ABR, and the earlier waves disappear first. If the audiogram is worse then 75 dB at 1000 and 2000 Hz, with no hearing at 4000 Hz, an ABR response for click stimuli of 95 dBnHL may not be obtained. Low frequency hearing loss does not have a significant effect on ABR parameters elicited by click.

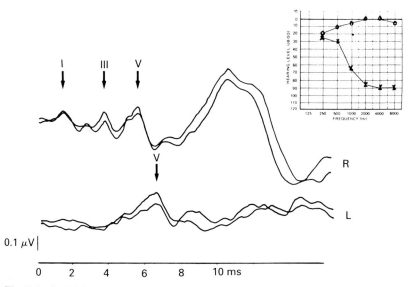

Fig. 7.2 An ABR recording in a case of cochlear hearing loss. Note that the earlier waves disappear before wave V.

Latency–intensity function

The latency of wave V decreases with increasing stimulus intensity. However, the latency–intensity function may not be parallel to normal slope. Cochlear hearing loss which demonstrates recruitment shows rapid latency changes with small increments of click intensity. The function of latency–intensity curves will be much steeper, as is shown in Figure 7.3.

In cases of predominantly high frequency, steep hearing loss, the latency–intensity function may have a shallow slope. This type of latency–intensity function can be explained by the fact that at high intensities the maximum contribution, normally coming from the 2000–4000 Hz region, is reduced in a case of high frequency hearing loss, and the initiation of the

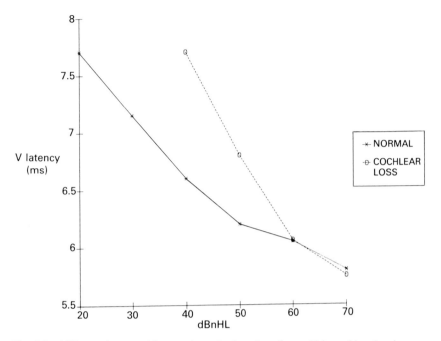

Fig. 7.3 ABR waveforms and latency–intensity function of wave V in cochlear hearing loss. The function is steeper than normal, and the change in waveform morphology can be seen.

ABR shifts to a more apically responding region in the cochlea. Therefore, the latency increases by the time necessary for the travelling wave to reach the responding region. On the other hand, initiation of ABR response to low intensity clicks shifts to the 1000–2000 Hz region, which is not affected in steep high frequency loss. An abnormally shallow latency–intensity function may suggest a high frequency hearing loss.

The diagnostic features indicating the type of hearing loss according to latency–intensity function are useful when present, but their absence has no diagnostic value. Clear differences between groups of patients with conductive and cochlear hearing loss can be demonstrated, but in individual cases the differentiation may be unreliable because of the complex interaction between stimulus intensity and various excitation patterns in the affected cochlea.

Effect of cochlear loss on ABR latencies

Several investigators have studied the effect of cochlear loss on latencies of ABR evoked by high intensity clicks. Wave V is the most prominent and most reliable in cochlear lesions, and, as a diagnostic parameter, it has become especially useful in differentiating cochlear from retrocochlear pathology.

Using 90 dBnHL clicks, Selters & Brackmann (1979) found that the latency of wave V is constant in hearing losses less than 50 dBnHL, but increases in greater losses. They empirically fitted a linear curve with 0.15 ms/10 dB of hearing loss, starting from 50 dB. Rosenhamer (1981) found latency increases of 0.1 ms/10 dB, starting at 30–40 dB of hearing loss. Hearing loss and age are interrelated, and they both have a complex effect on latency of wave V. A bivariate model of the effect of cochlear hearing loss and age on the latency of wave V has been suggested by Hyde (1985).

With 85 dBnHL clicks, the latency of wave V increases strongly and non-linearly with 4000 Hz pure-tone loss, and it also increases non-linearly with age, as shown in Figures 7.4 and 6.10. The non-linear latency behaviour is consistent with the notion that both ageing and cochlear hearing loss deplete a partially common cochlear population of responding units. Our data indicate that in patients with audiometric thresholds at 4000 Hz better than 50 dBnHL, the major variable accounting for inter-subject latency

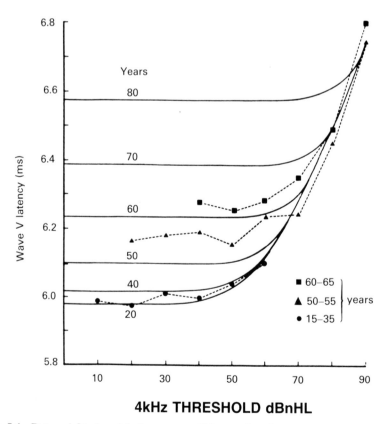

4kHz THRESHOLD dBnHL

Fig. 7.4 Data and fitted model of mean wave-V latency for effects of cochlear hearing loss (Abramovich & Hyde, unpublished).

variation is the age of the subject. For losses over 50 dB, the major contributing variable is hearing loss. For losses greater than 55 dB, there is a latency increase of 0.15 ms for every subsequent 10 dB of hearing loss. One can see at the bottom of Figure 7.4 that, for an age of about 20 years, the latency stays constant for small hearing losses and then goes up sharply as the loss exceeds 50 dBnHL. In elderly subjects, the latency of wave V starts off at higher values compared with young subjects, and does not begin to increase further until much larger hearing losses are encountered. If the age variable is not controlled, then the observed effect of hearing loss may vary in an unpredictable manner. Therefore, both hearing loss and age must be taken into account when interpreting ABR.

In symmetric cochlear hearing loss, the interaural latency difference among waves V (IT 5) has a standard deviation of about 0.2 ms.

The effect of audiometric contour has been studied by several authors. Jerger & Mauldin (1978) found that wave V latency correlates with the high frequency audiometric slope better than with the average audiometric hearing loss. With click stimuli, there is no evidence that low frequency hearing loss influences the latency of wave V. Rosenhamer (1981), Hyde (1985), and Abramovich (1987) have investigated a range of audiometric frequencies and audiometric slopes, using the partial correlation analysis method. It was found that the best correlation was with the hearing loss at 4000 Hz. The latency of wave V was not markedly affected by the slope of the audiogram.

The IPI I–V is a particularly stable parameter among the subjects. In cochlear hearing loss, IPI I–V is normal. The inter-peak interval IPI I–V is less sensitive to hearing loss than is wave V itself, and can contribute to a more accurate diagnosis. Eggermont et al (1980) studied the effect of unilateral pure-tone cochlear hearing loss, mainly in patients with Ménière's disease as compared with IPI I–V on the normal ear. The dominantly occurring differences in the I–V delays between both ears were 0 and 0.1 ms, with normal ears having a shorter latency.

The problem is that in many patients with cochlear hearing loss, especially at high frequencies, wave I is not identifiable using surface electrodes (Hyde & Blair 1981, Abramovich & Billings 1981). However, it has been reported (Coats 1978) that in the presence of high frequency hearing loss, IPI I–V can be reduced. This can be explained by the fact that at high stimulus intensities, the usual generation of wave I from the basal region shifts to a more apical region on the basilar membrane, where the hair cells are intact. This will delay wave I, and the I–V interval will shorten.

Estimation of hearing loss

The threshold can be estimated by reducing click intensity until the wave-V response is no longer reliably detected.

For flat audiometric contour, the sensitivity of click-evoked ABR is 10–15 dB, when relying on detection of wave V.

Be aware that in low frequency hearing loss, a normal, or near-normal click-evoked ABR can be recorded.

Changed excitation patterns and desynchronization in an affected cochlea, or much more so in the presence of a lesion in the brainstem, may reduce the response and affect the threshold estimation. Therefore, in order to justify using wave V as an index of peripheral hearing impairment, it is important to check the neurological criteria of ABR. If brain dysfunction is present, one should consider estimation of the threshold by detecting wave I, although its sensitivity is much less than that of wave V.

ABR IN MÉNIÈRE'S DISEASE

Pathophysiology

This has been described in Chapter 5. Schuknecht & Gulya (1983) have defined Ménière's disease as an expression of idiopathic, symptomatic endolymphatic hydrops. It is often found on autopsy that Reissner's membrane is distended to the walls of the scala vestibuli and that the saccular wall is distended to the footplate of the stapes (Schuknecht 1974). More recent work has stressed the effects of raised intracochlear pressure in this condition (Kanoh & Makimoto 1985, Tjernstrom & Casselbrant 1981).

Abnormalities of ABR

The ABR characteristics are similar to those in cochlear hearing loss. However, Parker & Thornton (1978) have shown how derived ABRs could be used to estimate travelling wave velocity (TWV). With this measurement, a novel application of ABR to the diagnosis of endolymphatic hydrops has been realized. The tentative hypothesis was that increased pressure in the scala media would lead to an increase in the stiffness of the basilar membrane, and, hence, the speed of the travelling wave along the basilar membrane would increase. The technique was applied to a 'definite' Ménière's disease group, and nearly all of the patients showed an increased TWV at high frequencies (Thornton et al 1989). Figure 7.5 shows an example.

The technique is too long for routine clinical application, and so a shortened form was developed for clinical use. This involves recording ABRs in response to click stimuli mixed with two different high-pass masking noises; it takes about 15 minutes. The latency difference of wave V, recorded in these two conditions, is compared with normal value. Too small a latency difference corresponds to an increased TWV and indicates raised endolym-

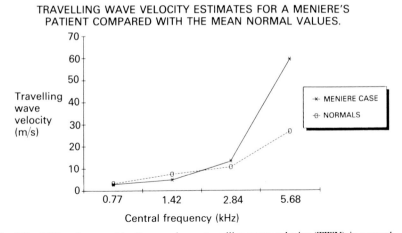

Fig. 7.5   ABR estimates of basilar membrane travelling wave velocity (TWV) in normal subjects and in a Ménière's disease patient.

phatic hydrops. This clinical technique has been verified (Thornton et al 1990) by monitoring Ménière's disease patients undergoing a glycerol dehydration procedure. All patients who showed an audiometric improvement also showed a TWV change relative to the normal value. Currently, this technique is undergoing clinical trials at Cambridge, Nottingham, and Southampton.

It seems probable that this test not only will enable those patients with increased endolymphatic pressure to be detected but also will enable the effects of drug treatment to be quickly and objectively monitored.

ABR IN VIIITH NERVE TUMOURS

Acoustic tumours comprise about 80% of cerebello-pontine angle tumours (Zulch 1957). Of 500 tumours diagnosed in Los Angeles, 95% were medium-sized or large (House 1979). However, there is a trend towards diagnosing smaller tumours, and in some studies 10% or more were detected when small (King & Morrison 1980, Nedzelski & Tator 1980).

The ABR test is proving to be a very important tool, and its performance in detecting acoustic tumours seems markedly superior to other tests in the traditional audiometric battery.

Pathophysiology of ABR

Large tumours may press and stretch the VIIIth nerve fibres as well as compress the brainstem. These factors may have an effect on neural transmission. It is thought that acoustic tumours cause a loss of neural synchronization in the affected population of nerve fibres, perhaps primarily

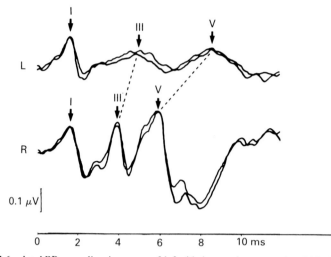

Fig. 7.6 An ABR recording in a case of left-sided acoustic tumour in which the distal part of the nerve is intact. This leaves a normal wave I, but with peaks III and V delayed and reduced in amplitude. (From Journal of Laryngology and Otology 1987, 101: 336, with permission.)

in the high-frequency fibres on the exterior of the nerve, probably causing also a minor increase in conduction delay (Eggermont et al 1980).

Eggermont et al (1980) found that the IPI I–V, recorded using narrow-band stimuli, was borderline normal, but that the overall I–V delay in stimulation with broad-band click was abnormal. They concluded that this was due to the desynchronizing effect of the tumour on the high-frequency fibres. This leads to elimination, depression, or delay of ABR waves generated at more rostral sites. When the distal part of the nerve is intact, it generates wave I, representing mainly neural activity of the high-frequency fibres. Such a tumour record is shown in Figure 7.6. A larger, extracanalicular, acoustic neuroma can obliterate all waves following wave I (Fig. 7.7).

When the tumour presses on the brainstem, an abnormal ABR may be recorded on the contralateral side as well (Fig. 7.8). It has been proposed that this is due to compression of the brainstem at the level of the superior olive, which is thought to be responsible for generation of wave III from the opposite side (Rudge 1983, Musiek et al 1987).

Diagnostic parameters of ABR

The ABR waveforms and latency measures for differential diagnosis between cochlear and retrocochlear lesions are obtained by stimulating each ear with high-intensity clicks. Diagnostic ABR features include abnormal ABR wave morphology and abnormal amplitudes, but the most important parameters used in the detection of acoustic tumours are the absolute

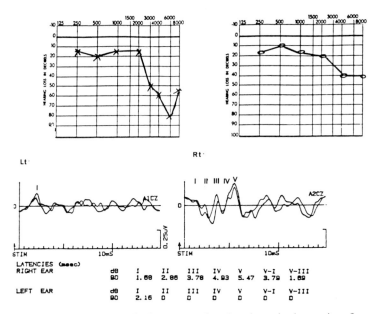

LATENCIES (msec)									
RIGHT EAR	dB	I	II	III	IV	V		V-I	V-III
	80	1.68	2.86	3.78	4.93	5.47		3.79	1.69
LEFT EAR	dB	I	II	III	IV	V		V-I	V-III
	80	2.16	0	0	0	0		0	0

Fig. 7.7   From a larger extracanalicular tumour than that shown in the previous figure. In this case, waves III and V cannot be seen. The ABR was crucial in leading to a CT scan and the final diagnosis.

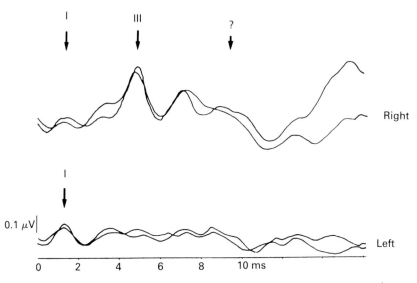

Fig. 7.8   ABR recordings from patient with a large left-sided acoustic tumour pressing on the brainstem.

latency of wave V (LV), the inter-peak interval between waves I, III, and V (IPI I–III, I–V), and the interaural latency difference among waves V (IT 5).

The waveform should be inspected for abnormal or absent waves III and V and for a 50% reversal in the V/I amplitude ratio from expected normal ratio.

Waveforms and amplitudes of ABR

Common results in proven acoustic tumours are a loss of all waves except wave I, and delay and depression of waves which come from sites rostral to the tumour, especially wave V. Small acoustic tumours that are clearly extrinsic and without brainstem compression can produce abnormal waves III and V. Figure 7.6 shows a typical tumour record, with a normal wave I, but with waves III and V flattened and delayed. Increase in I–V interval is the critical diagnostic feature. In tumour cases, wave V is more frequently identifiable than is wave III.

In tumours with considerable high-frequency hearing loss, wave I can be eliminated, and only the more prominent (but delayed) wave V may be detected (Fig. 7.9). In many cases of tumour, wave V is not merely delayed, but absent (Fig. 7.10). If wave I is still present, this is a very strong indication of a tumour.

A wave V/wave I amplitude ratio of less than 1 is considered abnormal;

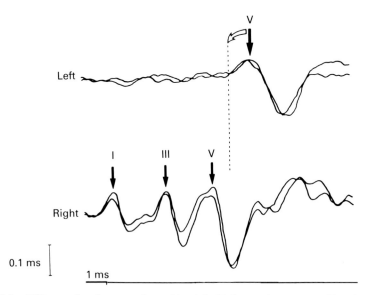

Fig. 7.9   ABR recording from a patient with a left-sided acoustic tumour, with only wave V present on the affected side.

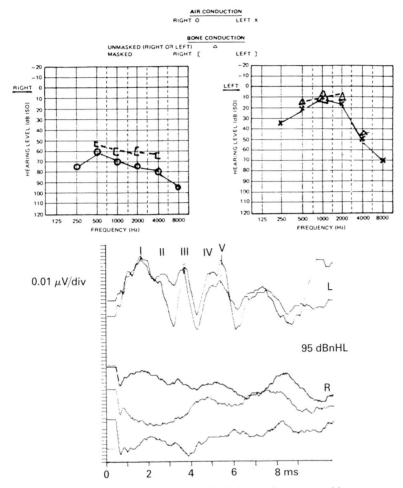

Fig. 7.10 ABR recording in a patient with left-sided acoustic tumour, with no response on the affected side. Note that the hearing threshold in the left ear was 70 dBnHL.

however, this is not a reliable diagnostic parameter for acoustic tumours. High-frequency hearing loss can reduce markedly the amplitude of wave I, and it can thus become a confounding factor in the interpretation of the V/I ratio.

The diagnostic significance of an absence of ABR has limited specificity. If the hearing loss is not severe, then response absence is the most extreme case of response delay, and the finding is strongly indicative of a tumour. As noted in Chapter 6, at some point, hearing loss of cochlear origin eliminates the ABR, and the value of the finding is lost. Technical error and idiopathic ABR absence are also possibilities. It should be noted that the proportion of absent ABRs obtained in any study will depend strongly upon the patterns and severity of hearing losses included in the study. In a study by Barrs et al (1985), ABRs were absent in 37% of patients with acoustic tumours.

ABR abnormalities in acoustic tumours are usually on the ipsilateral side, but abnormal changes on the contralateral side may occur when the brainstem is compressed or axially shifted by a big tumour (see Fig. 7.8). Therefore, it is important to record from both sides, even when there is severe unilateral hearing loss, and ABR may not be recorded from the affected ear.

The pattern of ABR abnormalities has been studied by Josey et al (1984). In 181 patients with surgically confirmed, internal, auditory-canal and cerebello-pontine angle tumours, the following abnormalities were observed in tumorous ears: there were no identifiable waves on ABR in 72 ears, only wave I was seen in 9 ears, the only identifiable and prolonged wave V latency was observed in 46 ears, and prolongation of inter-peak intervals was seen in 50 patients; only 5 patients had normal traces.

Latency of wave V

Some early cases of acoustic tumour waveform can give approximately normal ABR, and the only abnormality may be prolongation of the latencies of the late waves. Generally, prolongation of waves III and V is an important diagnostic feature.

The various diagnostic ABR features vary in sensitivity, specificity, and ease of measurement. For example, 20–38% of tumour suspects were reported to have a prolongation of latency of wave V falsely suggestive of retrocochlear involvement (Clemis & McGee 1979, Abramovich & Billings 1981). The major cause for this is increase of latency of wave V due to cochlear hearing loss, though age and other sources of variation among subjects contribute to errors.

Selters & Brackmann (1979) applied a wave-V latency correction factor based on the pure-tone hearing loss at 4000 Hz. For hearing losses greater than 50 dB, they used a correction factor and subtracted from absolute latency V value, 0.10 ms/10 dB for further hearing losses. According to them, for example, for a hearing loss of 80 dB at 4000 Hz on the audiogram, the correction factor is 0.3 ms. This reduces their false-positive rate from 24 to 8%, but they stress that the chance of error increases with 4000 Hz losses above 75 dB.

Because ABR diagnostic error rates depend on latency correction for hearing loss, the effect of hearing loss and age has been investigated, and a bivariate model for latency correction used, as shown in Figure 7.4 (Hyde 1985, Abramovich 1988). The results of the model suggest that when correcting the ABR wave V latencies for tumour investigation, both hearing loss and age must be taken into account. With the start at 55 dB, the correction factor is about 0.15 ms for every 10 dB of hearing loss.

Interaural latency difference of wave V (IT 5)

The interaural latency difference of wave V (IT 5) is more specific than the absolute latency of wave V, because the non-tumorous ear acts as a partial control for age and sex. Selters & Brackmann (1977) investigated patients with various degrees of cochlear hearing loss and derived a nomogram. They found that for losses at 4000 Hz up to 60 dBnHL, the interaural latency difference was less than 0.2 ms; for losses of 60 dB to 75 dB, less than 0.3 ms; and for greater losses, less than 0.4 ms. These criteria enabled them to separate cochlear losses from tumours, the latter having a longer interaural latency difference.

If the IT 5 criterion of greater than 0.2 ms is used for tumour detection, then a very high false-positive rate can occur, 25% being reported in suspects by Bauch et al (1982). It should be noted that the false-positive rate obtained in any study depends greatly upon the pattern and severity of hearing loss included in the study sample. Some investigators advise that an IT 5 greater than 0.3 ms is significant and may indicate a retrocochlear lesion (Terkildsen et al 1981). In hearing losses greater than 65 dB, a 0.4 ms–IT 5 criterion has been applied by Clemis & McGee (1979).

Although the unaffected ear acts as a partial control for age and sex, IT 5 is still subject to the major variable of hearing loss. Selters & Brackmann (1979) reduced the false-positive rate from 24 to 8% by correcting LV of the affected ear for hearing loss. After correction, the difference of more than 0.2 ms was suggestive of a tumour and was used as a diagnostic criterion. The detection rate was 92.7%.

Some investigators showed that the magnitude of the interaural wave V latency difference is related to the size of the tumour (Selters & Brackmann 1979); however, in individual cases this is not always so (Eggermont et al 1980). In very large tumours that press against the brainstem, an increase in wave V latency may be found on stimulating the non-tumorous ear. This may decrease the interaural latency delay IT 5 (Rudge 1985).

Figure 7.9 shows an example of latency correction; there are normal ABR waves from the right ear, and from the left ear one can see only delayed wave V. The patient had a severe hearing loss: was the wave V delay attributable to cochlear loss, or was there a tumour? The open arrow and dotted line show the latency correction by our model. This reduces the delay, but there is still enough of a difference between the ears to diagnose a tumour, a diagnosis which was correct.

Both age and hearing loss must be taken into consideration in using IT 5 criterion. When properly corrected for loss and age in the above manner, IT 5 gives a lower than 5% false-positive error rate, with the IT 5 criterion of 0.3 ms (Abramovich 1987). Low false-positive rates are desirable; however, this must be weighed carefully against the possible increases in the false-negative rate. Using an IT 5 criterion of 0.2 ms, Barrs et al (1985) found a false-negative rate of 2% in 229 patients with proven acoustic tumours.

Inter-peak intervals (IPI I–V)

Prolongation of intervals I–III and I–V is a common feature in acoustic tumours. When all waves are present, the I–III interval is reported to be more affected than III–V, although the reverse is possible (Fig. 7.11). In very large tumours that press against the brainstem, an increase in the wave III–V delay is found when stimulating the non-tumorous ear.

IPI I–V is less sensitive to hearing loss than wave V itself, and it is normal in conductive and cochlear hearing losses, but prolonged in retrocochlear disorders (Fig. 7.12). The IPI I–V delay in cases of acoustic tumour appears to relate to tumour size, and increasing tumour size results in larger IPI I–V delays, according to data in Eggermont et al (1980). The mean value of IPI I–V is approximately 4 ms, with a standard deviation (SD) of about 0.2 ms, giving a 95% confidence limit of the mean value plus 0.4 ms. Greater values should be regarded as suggestive of acoustic tumour.

Few false-negative results have been reported (Rosenhamer 1977, Selters & Brackmann 1977, Clemis & McGee 1979, Eggermont et al 1980, Djupesland et al 1981). Portmann et al (1980) pointed out that IPI I–V delays greater than 4.5 ms suggest a tumour. A detection rate of 95% with 5% false-positive results was reported by Eggermont et al (1980), who used IPI I–V criterion of 4.33 ms (mean value of 4.01 ms plus 2 SD of 0.16 ms). When the IPI I–V criterion for tumour detection was greater than 4.49 ms (mean plus 3 SD), the ABR test missed 10% of the cases with no false-positive results.

The non-affected ear can be used as a partial control, and, according to Eggermont et al (1980), it is unlikely that in cases of cochlear hearing loss, IPI I–V differ by more than 0.4 ms.

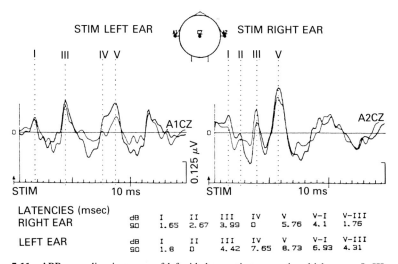

Fig. 7.11 ABR recording in a case of left-sided acoustic tumour in which waves I, III, and V can be recorded. Note prolongation of the intervals I–III and I–V, with near normal amplitudes.

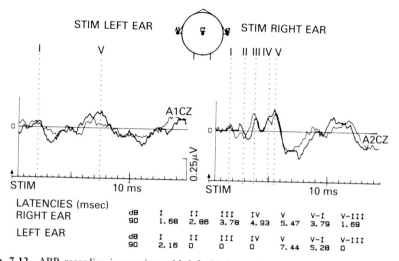

Fig. 7.12 ABR recording in a patient with left-sided acoustic tumour. Note prolongation of I–V interval. Wave III is difficult to identify.

Combined IPI I–V and IT 5 measures

ABR testing has been reported to be an excellent test for acoustic-tumour detection, being positive in 90–100% of confirmed cases (Rosenhamer 1977, Selters & Brackmann 1979, Clemis & McGee 1979, Eggermont et al 1980, Portmann et al 1980, Terkildsen et al 1981, Djupesland et al 1981, Bauch et al 1982, Cashman & Rossman 1983, Barrs et al 1985).

The various diagnostic features vary in sensitivity, specificity, and ease of measurement. Depending on which diagnostic parameters are used, the false-positive error rate may vary from about 30 to about 5% (Clemis & McGee 1979, Bauch et al 1982, Selters & Brackmann 1979, Eggermont et al 1980, Terkildsen et al 1981, Abramovich 1987).

Accurate pure-tone audiometry is desirable prior to ABR testing and interpretation, especially if good control of false-positive errors of LV and IT 5 by a latency correction method is required. The ABR measure of IPI I–V is less sensitive to the effects of hearing loss than LV or IT 5, and can contribute to a more accurate overall interpretation. However, in 30 to 60% of patients with cochlear hearing loss, and in most cases with severe high-frequency hearing loss, wave I is not identifiable in ABR records with surface electrodes (Abramovich & Billings 1981, Hyde & Blair 1981). Here we must rely on LV and IT 5, or, alternatively, wave I generated from the cochlear nerve can be revealed by transtympanic or endomeatal electrocochleography.

Combining IPI I–V and IT 5 further improves the detection rate with very small false-positive rates. In a few cases, responses may be normal for one of the parameters but abnormal for others. The combination of both parameters can augment the detection rate by using even more stringent criteria (Eggermont et al 1980).

ABR IN CEREBELLO-PONTINE (CP)-ANGLE LESIONS

ABR in CP-angle tumours

Pathology

Tumours which are not attached to the VIIIth nerve may grow to a large size before exerting pressure and stretching the VIIIth nerve, as well as compressing the brainstem and producing an effect similar to that of an acoustic tumour (Chiappa 1983). These are less common CP-angle tumours such as petrous ridge and tentorial meningiomas, lower cranial nerve neurofibromas, gliomas, cholesteatomas, and others.

ABR findings

The IPI can be prolonged considerably, for example, in CP-angle meningiomas, and wave I is preserved in the majority of cases (Fig. 7.13). Any ABR abnormality found on the side contralateral to the tumour is attributed to brainstem displacement.

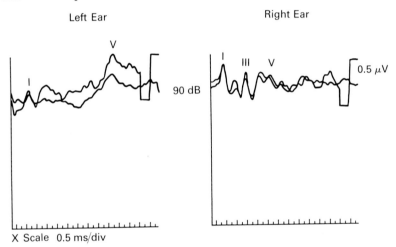

Fig. 7.13   ABR recording in a patient with a large CP-angle meningioma. Note preservation of wave I and prolongation of the interval I–V.

ABR in vascular lesions of CP angle

Pathology

Aneurysms in the cerebello-pontine angle can cause similar effects to those of tumours by exerting pressure on the nerve and the brainstem.

ABR findings

Johnson & Kline (1978) reported abnormal ABR in cases of aneurysms of the anterior inferior cerebellar artery. Bilateral ABR abnormalities were demonstrated in a case of right-sided basilar artery aneurysm in the posterior fossa with displacement of the fourth ventricle. This aneurysm caused low-frequency hearing loss on the audiogram (Musiek et al 1987). The early waves I and II on the right side and waves I, II, and III on the left side were normal, but the subsequent waves were absent. The authors explained that the lesion exerted its main effect not on the cochlear nerve, but on the cochlear nucleus and superior olivary complex. This pattern of ABR is similar to and consistent with the contralateral effect caused by a tumour.

Vascular compression of the VIIth and adjacent VIIIth nerves by the loop of the anterior inferior cerebellar artery has been suggested as the cause of hemifacial spasm, and sometimes of associated changes in ABR resulting in increase of IPI III–V (Moller et al 1982). In this study, abnormal ABR for both ipsilateral and contralateral sides were observed in trigeminal neuralgia. The authors explained bilateral changes in ABR as being due to vascular loops of the anterior inferior cerebellar artery and sometimes superior cerebellar arteries pressing on the Vth nerve and lower brainstem in the region of the cochlear nucleus or trapezoid body. Because the auditory fibres cross at this level to the opposite side, ABR changes on the contralateral side can be expected.

ABR in infections of the VIIIth nerve

Pathology

Abnormal ABRs have been reported in some patients with Ramsay Hunt syndrome who exhibited facial palsy, vesicular eruption, and auditory-vestibular symptoms (Abramovich & Prasher 1986). Acute inflammation of the neural and perineural structures of the VIIth and adjacent VIIIth nerves, and possibly of the surface of the brain-stem, was caused by the neurotropic virus *Varicella zoster*, which could also be a factor in the underlying process of desynchronization and poor conduction.

ABR findings

The ABRs may result in prolonged inter-peak intervals of the ABR components and in abnormalities of wave morphology. The striking feature of the abnormalities in these patients was the prolongation of the latencies of waves III and V, with preservation of wave I, which clearly suggests retrocochlear involvement. In all patients tested, the abnormalities were on the affected side (Fig. 7.14). When the patients were retested 6 months later, after clinical recovery, the ABRs appeared within normal limits.

ABR IN BRAINSTEM LESIONS

Brainstem, cerebello-pontine angle, and VIIIth nerve involvement can result in similar abnormalities of the ABR, making differentiation difficult. The

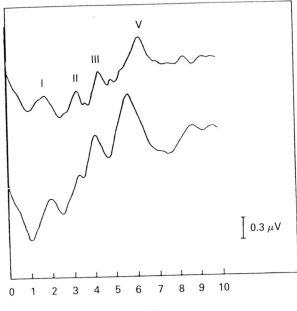

Time (ms)

Fig. 7.14 ABR recordings in a patient with Ramsay Hunt syndrome (*Varicella zoster* virus infection). Abnormally prolonged waves III and V appear on affected side (lower trace), although the hearing is normal (15 dBnHL at 4000 Hz). Normal ABR responses from unaffected side are on upper trace. (From Archives of Otolaryngology 1986, 112: 927.)

abnormalities of particular brainstem components may also be due to a lesion at the site of a generator or at the level preceding it, as indicated by studies of specific brainstem lesions (Chiappa & Yiannikas 1983). However, some common features can suggest the level of the lesion in the brainstem. The most valuable ABR parameters for detection of neurological impairment are prolonged inter-peak intervals among waves I, III, and V.

Lesions in the high levels of the brainstem can produce ipsilateral, bilateral, and, to a lesser extent, contralateral abnormalities. The presence of earlier ABR components with prolonged IPI III–V or absent later waves usually suggests a lesion in the upper part of the brainstem.

Lesions of the lower brainstem more often produce unilateral ABR abnormalities, unless the lesion is large.

Tumours

Pathophysiology of ABR

Tumours affecting the brainstem can be visualized as originating either inside the brainstem or outside but close to the brainstem. The former type of tumours are called intrinsic, and the latter are called extrinsic.

Tumours outside the brainstem may exert pressure that distorts or extends into the brainstem to produce an abnormal ABR.

The ABR does not reveal the nature of the tumour, or indicate whether it is an intrinsic or extrinsic lesion. However, some clinical correlations of the tumour site and the ABR have clarified possible patterns of wave abnormalities.

ABR abnormalities

For example, the tumours originating from the cerebello-pontine angle may produce changes in the ABR similar to those of lower brainstem involvement.

Extrinsic tumours originating from the cerebellum, meningiomas of the tentorium, pineal gland tumours, and aneurysms can produce ABR changes compatible with upper brainstem lesions. The ABR can appear normal until late in the course of the disease in intrinsic brainstem tumours; Rudge (1983) observed remarkably normal ABR in a number of ambulant patients.

A midbrain lesion may be detected by a prolongation of the IPIs. Figure 7.15 shows such a case, in which the I–III interval is normal, but the III–V interval is extended. The contralateral responses are all normal.

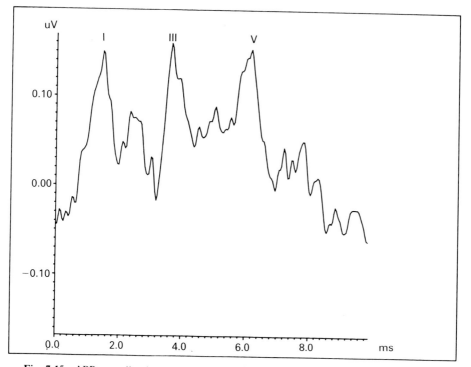

Fig. 7.15 ABR recording in a patient with a midbrain lesion. Note prolongation of the III–V interval.

An astrocytoma of the lower and upper brainstem, extending from the left medullo-pontine region up to the left inferior colliculus, was shown to have eliminated the waves rostral to wave I, on stimulating the left side, in an example given by Starr & Hamilton (1976). On stimulating the right ear, they found all ABR waves to be present on that side; however, the amplitude of the IV/V complex was depressed and the V/I ratio was abnormally reduced by 50%. Big extrinsic cerebello-pontine angle tumours may cause similar ABR changes.

Prolongation and depression of wave V with an abnormal V/I amplitude ratio in upper brainstem tumours can be recorded. This pattern has been reported in unilateral midbrain tumours after stimulating the opposite ear.

In a large upper brainstem tumour, for example, pineal germinoma in the midbrain region and rostral pontine tegmen, as described by Starr & Hamilton (1976), the ABR showed no waves IV, V, or VI on either side. The slight prolongation of wave II and III was explained as a secondary effect of pressure from the tumour.

Multiple sclerosis and other demyelinating diseases

Pathology

The factors responsible for demyelination in the nerve fibres could be due to an abnormal autoimmune response, induced by virus, toxins, trauma, or inherited leucodystrophies. Demyelination is characterized by perivascular oedema, infiltration by lymphocytes and monocytes, glial cell proliferation, and subsequent scarring. It is thought that partial remyelination is possible, but deficient.

Demyelination reduces the speed of conduction and the ability to transmit stimuli at fast-repetition rates, producing latency delays of the ABR. Also, the reduced synchrony results in degradation of the ABR. Involvement of the myelin of the VIIIth nerve is not uncommon in the presence of the normal hearing threshold (Jacobson et al 1986).

ABR abnormalities

Clinically, multiple sclerosis (MS) is characterized by exacerbation and remission of symptoms, and it is classified as definite, probable, or possible (McAlpine et al 1972, Bauer 1980). Patients with clinical evidence of a brainstem lesion at the time of recording have a higher proportion of ABR abnormalities than do those who do not show brainstem disorder (Robinson & Rudge 1977). Abnormal ABRs were found in 75% of definite, 33% of probable, and 29% of possible MS patients in a study by Lynn et al (1980). The implication is that ABR analysis can detect clinically silent lesions, and therefore that it is very sensitive, but, of course, in detecting lesions in MS it will detect only those cases in which there is brainstem involvement.

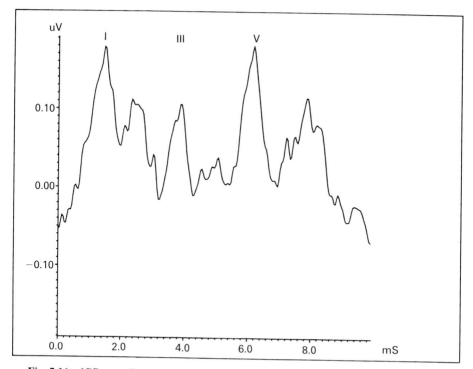

Fig. 7.16 ABR recording in a MS patient with generalized brainstem lesion. The intervals I–III, III–V and I–V are all prolonged.

The ABR abnormalities include increased inter-peak intervals, decrease of the amplitudes and V/I ratios, absence of peaks, and poor waveform reproducibility. Figure 7.16 illustrates a case.

Waveform and amplitude of ABR

Most ABR abnormalities are related to wave V. Low amplitude of, or even absence of, wave V was seen in as much as 87% of abnormal ABRs in the patients with MS studied by Chiappa (1983), and in patients with normal latencies, 50% were found with abnormally reduced wave-V amplitude by Robinson & Rudge (1975).

The amplitudes of all main peaks may be reduced or even absent, and the repeatability of the response in retested MS patients is poor compared to normal subjects (Prasher & Gibson 1980, Robinson & Rudge 1980).

Latencies of ABR

In a high proportion of ABR abnormalities in MS, decreased amplitude values, as well as latency increases, occur. Figure 7.17 shows the amplitude–

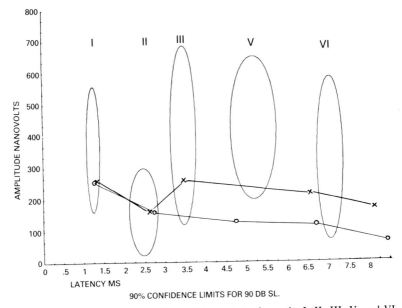

Fig. 7.17   The amplitude–latency 90% confidence limits for peaks I, II, III, V, and VI. The left-side results show normal values for peaks I–III, and increased latencies for peaks V and VI. The right-side results show increased latencies for peaks III, V, and VI, and significant decreases in the amplitude.

latency 90% confidence limits for peaks I, II, III, V, and VI. The left-side results from an MS patient show normal values for peaks I–III and increased latencies for peaks V and VI. The right-side results show increased latencies for peaks III, V, and VI, and significant decreases in amplitude. Delay in the latency of wave I is much less common, and it suggests involvement of the distal part of the VIIIth nerve (Jacobson et al 1986).

Occasionally, contralateral stimulation alone results in abnormal prolongation of the latencies, and, therefore, it has been suggested that contralateral recording should be used in neuro-otological testing in order to increase the detection rate of brainstem lesion (Prasher & Gibson 1980, Quaranta et al 1986).

Stressing the auditory system by increasing the stimulation rate from 10 to 80/s results in abnormal prolongation of the IPI and some increase in the identification of MS (Robinson & Rudge 1977).

A combination of abnormal parameters of the ABR is common, and Barajas (1982) reported that in 25% of all detected ABR abnormalities the IPIs alone were abnormal, in 45% the amplitude of wave V was abnormal, and in 30% both abnormalities were present.

Vascular lesions

Pathophysiology

Brainstem vascular disturbances can manifest themselves as degenerative arterial disease or as migraine, and changes in the vertebrobasilar arterial system can compromise oxygenation of the brainstem. Cochlear hearing loss can also be associated with degenerative vascular disease.

ABR findings

Absolute latency of wave V and IPI I–V can be prolonged in vertebrobasilar lesions. The amplitude ratio of wave V to wave I also can be abnormal, i.e. less than 1.

In general, patients with transient ischaemic attacks of brainstem structures have normal ABR, unless there are permanent deficits (Chiappa 1983).

If there is a brainstem infarct, the ABR will be abnormal when the infarct involves the auditory pathway. The incidence of abnormal ABR in patients with brainstem infarction is very high; it has been reported by some investigators in 100% of cases (Starr & Hamilton 1976, Hashimoto et al 1979). Ragazzoni et al (1982) studied ABR in patients with vertebrobasilar reversible ischaemic attacks, and reported an increase in inter-peak latencies. Abnormal I–V intervals were reported by Rosenhall et al (1981) in 36 out of 48 patients with vertebrobasilar arterial system disorders. Rudge (1985) used a binaural stimulation strategy to test ambulant patients with vascular brainstem disturbance who were not in an acute phase. He found abnormalities in 20% of the patients. However, in a group of patients with more severe disabilities, ABR abnormalities were more frequent.

Infections

Pathology

Most perinatal infections associated with hearing loss cause an inner-ear rather than a central-hearing disorder. Cochlear hearing loss in meningitis may be a result of vasculitis of the inner-ear vessels. A secondary fibrous reaction with adhesions following meningitis may be associated with VIIIth nerve dysfunction (Friedmann 1974). CNS hearing abnormalities can be reversible, and the changes may be related to vasculitis and transiently raised intracranial pressure.

ABR findings

Prolonged inter-peak intervals I–III have been recorded in some cases of bacterial and viral meningitis (Chiappa 1983). The abnormal IPI usually reverts to normal (Hecox et al 1981).

Abnormal waveforms, reduced amplitudes of the IV/V complex, and prolonged IPI I–III and III–V have been found in patients with brainstem encephalitis. ABR resolution paralleled clinical improvement (Rosenblatt & Majnemer 1984).

Normal ABRs have been reported in postinfectious, subacute, sclerosing panencephalitis (Chiappa 1983).

Neurological disorders

Abnormal ABRs were reported in a proportion of patients with various neurodegenerative disorders, inherited neuropathies, inherited demyelinating metabolic disturbances, chromosomal disorders, and structural malformations (Rudge 1983, Chiappa 1983, Hecox 1985). Deterioration in ABR usually is noticed with neurological progression of the disorder but adds little to the diagnosis (Hecox 1985).

Head trauma

ABRs have been recorded in patients with severe head injury, and various patterns have been observed including, normal, prolonged IPI; the absence of waves V and III; and no response (Tsubokawa et al 1980, Brewer & Resnick 1984). Loss of all waves or those proximal to wave I carried a prognosis of death or persistent vegetative state.

8. Middle-latency responses (MLR)

INTRODUCTION

Middle-latency responses (MLR) recorded from the scalp have latencies in the range 10–50 ms. Some of the potentials are of myogenic origin, and most respond only to relatively high-intensity acoustic stimuli. However, the postauricular muscle response (PAM) has a relatively low threshold (Thornton 1975). Middle-latency neurogenic potentials are thought to originate in the thalamus and its primary projections, and possibly in the primary cortex.

Neurogenic middle-latency responses have some value in audiometric threshold estimation, especially for low frequencies. They also offer a useful supplementary test in neuro-otology for the detection of brainstem disorder, for example, in multiple sclerosis and tumours.

GENERATORS OF MIDDLE-LATENCY RESPONSES

The middle-latency responses in man were described as long ago as 1958 by Geisler et al, and they have been studied by Goldstein & Rodman (1967) and Mendel & Goldstein (1969). Initially, they were called 'early' responses. However, they were renamed 'middle-latency responses' soon after the discovery of ABRs, which were classified as early-latency responses (Davis 1976).

Both myogenic and neurogenic potentials occur in the time domain when the stimulus is of high intensity (Bickford et al 1964, Picton et al 1974). However, for low- and moderate-intensity sounds, there is substantial evidence of the neural origin of middle-latency response (Maast 1965). At least a partly neural origin of middle-latency response has been confirmed in the induction of muscle paralysis during anaesthesia. Wave morphology similar to MLR was obtained by Harker et al (1977), as was Pa potential by Kileny et al (1983).

The sites of MLR generators have not yet been determined with certainty, but for the earlier MLR components No, Po, and Na, the medial geniculate ganglion and the thalamus have been suggested (Davis 1976). Generation of No, Po, and Na or SN10 has also been attributed to postsynaptic activity from the inferior colliculus in man (Hashimoto 1982). Evidence has been given for a primary cortical origin of a middle-latency auditory-evoked potential in laboratory animals, e.g. cats (Kaga et al 1980, Buchwald et al 1981). However, in man there is some uncertainty whether MLR components arise in the primary cortex. Parving et al (1980) also observed normal Pa in patients with auditory agnosia due to temporal lobe lesion. Kraus et al (1982) also observed normal Na and Pa in patients with unilateral temporal lobe lesion, but found elimination or reduction of the amplitudes in patients with bitemporal lesions. Also, generators of the Na component are more effectively activated by contralateral stimulation (Woods & Clayworth 1985).

The post-auricular muscle response was first reported by Kiang et al (1963), who described it as a variable low-threshold response. Douek et al (1973) stressed the importance of recording from both sides simultaneously, as the response has a bilateral representation. Picton et al (1974) reported that the PAM response was highly variable, both within and among subjects.

METHODS

MLR

Testing environment

Neurogenic MLRs are recorded in a testing environment similar to that of ABR. They are tested in awake, passively co-operative patients.

Electrode placement

Non-polarizing silver/silver chloride electrodes are used. The optimal sites for the active pair of electrodes are the vertex Cz and periauricular region A1 or A2. The earth electrode is placed on the forehead at Fz or on the contralateral mastoid.

Technical aspects of stimulation and MLR recording

In order to elicit MLRs, a good neural synchrony is required, which can be achieved by using rapid rise-time stimuli. Usually stimuli click are presented monaurally as an electrical pulse of 100 μs duration through an electrodynamic transducer. For tone bursts, a 2 ms duration rise–fall and plateau are used most often in clinical practice. In order to estimate the hearing threshold, 256–1024 sweeps are taken at varying intensities for reliable identification of the peaks. Since the MLR occurs within 100-ms intervals, the repetition rate should be below 10 stimuli/s in order to avoid superimposition of the response.

However, it was found that when using stimulation rate of 40/s (40 Hz), the main peaks become superimposed, interfere constructively, and produce a sinusoidal response (Galambos et al 1981). This '40-Hz' MLR response can be used for threshold estimation (see Fig. 8.1).

A commonly used band-pass filter for acquisition of the MLR is 30–300 Hz. The analysis time for the MLR record is 100 ms.

PAM response

Testing environment

Because this is a myogenic response, the response amplitude is dependent upon muscle tone. If the patient is lying in bed, the response may be enhanced by using pillows to push the head forward, thus increasing muscle tone in the postauricular region. For this reason, this response may be the easiest to record in active children. Good responses are also obtained when a child is held on its mother's lap.

Electrode placement

PAM is a near-field response and the active electrode is placed on the mastoid process over the postauricular muscle, with the indifferent electrode at Cz and the earth at Fz. The position of the indifferent and earth electrodes is not critical.

Technical aspects of stimulation and PAM recording

Click stimuli are used, and generally some 200–300 presentations are required to obtain a clear response waveform. A window of at least 30 ms should be used in order to record all the peaks of the response. A stimulation rate of approximately 10 clicks/s, whilst adapting the response somewhat, provides a good compromise in minimizing the recording times in the clinic. Thornton (1975) investigated the effects of recording bandwidths and showed that a bandwidth from 100 to 3000 Hz is required to obtain all the components of the response.

NORMATIVE CHARACTERISTICS OF MLR

Waveform

A criterion for the interpretation of the MLR is its waveform morphology. The MLR consists of a number of negative and positive peaks identified, according to nomenclature, as No, Po, Na, Pa, Nb, and Pb (Fig. 8.1). It is thought that No is synonymous with wave V. However, not all subjects show all components. The most reliable component is Na–Pa, and it is used

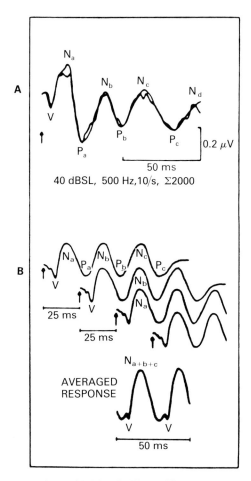

Fig. 8.1 (**A**) Normal waveform of MLR. (**B**) The 40-Hz response which comprises the 'in-phase' addition of MLRs. (Reproduced with permission from Galambos et al 1981.)

to estimate the hearing threshold. The early No component is identical with the SN10 wave of the brainstem response, and the late Pb component is analogous to the P1 early component of the cortical response.

Amplitude and intensity–amplitude relationship

The amplitudes are prone to considerable variations among subjects, and the most reliable is the measurement of Na–Pa amplitude, which is about 0.5–2 μV. Greater amplitudes are seen in response to 500 Hz tone bursts, as compared to 2000 and 4000 Hz tone bursts. The amplitude of the MLR increases with increasing stimulus intensity up to 60 dBnHL, after which the effect is less noticeable (Ozdamar & Kraus 1983).

Latency and intensity–latency relationship

The latency of MLR has not been accepted as a useful diagnostic parameter, because of its considerable inter-subject variability. The latencies of the peaks of the components vary within the following ranges: No, 8–10 ms; Po, 10–13 ms; Na, 16–30 ms; Pa, 30–45 ms; Nb, 40–50 ms; and Pb, 55–80 ms. In response to tone bursts, the latencies tend to decrease as frequency is increased (McFarland et al 1977). The latencies decrease slightly with increase of stimulus intensity (Mendel 1974).

40-Hz MLR

Galambos et al (1981) noticed that the main negative peaks Na and Nb of MLR are at approximately 25 and 50 ms, respectively. By stimulating at 25-ms intervals, which corresponds to frequency of 40 Hz, they showed that the amplitude of the response increased to approximately twice that of the MLR obtained by stimulating at a rate of 10/s (see Fig. 8.1).

PAM response

As the PAM is a vestigial response, it is not found in all normal subjects. However, when a response is obtained there are two mastoid negative peaks at approximately 12 and 18 ms, respectively, with positive peaks at 15 and 22 ms (Thornton 1975). Figure 8.2 shows a typical response at various stimulus levels.

FACTORS INFLUENCING NORMAL MLR

Age

In neonates at term, the most consistent components proved to be Po and Na, and the latencies decreased significantly in the first 3 months (Rotteveel et al 1986). The later peaks Nb and Pb are difficult to see in children (Okitsu 1984). The detectability of both Na and Pa increases significantly as a function of age, and by 10–14 years of age, these components are similar to those found in adults; they have been found in 100% of cases (Kraus et al 1985, Suzuki & Hirabayashi 1987). The absence of MLR in younger children should not be taken as an indication of hearing loss.

Effect of sleep and anaesthetic agents

The MLR in sleep differ from those in the wakening state, especially in children, and considerable decrease in detectability of Pa was found in sleep (Okitsu 1984). The 40 Hz MLR response is also reduced during sleep.

Following induction of anaesthesia using volatile anaesthetics such as halothane or enflurane, the latencies of Na and Nb increase; and the

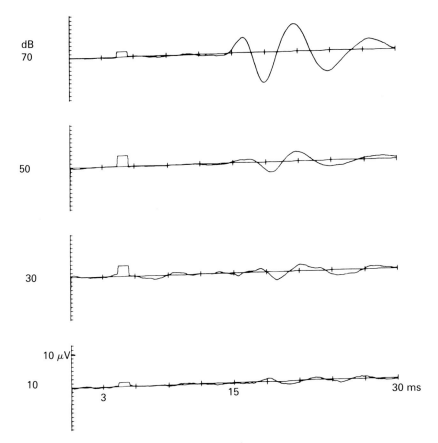

Fig. 8.2   PAM responses at various stimulus levels.

amplitudes considerably decrease with increasing concentration of the agents (Thornton et al 1984) (Fig. 8.3).

Sedation and anaesthesia interfere with the muscle tone which is required for PAM response.

Effect of masking

Gutnick & Goldstein (1978) considered the MLR suitable as an audiometric tool, and did not find the MLR affected by contralateral masking.

FREQUENCY SPECIFICITY AND THRESHOLD ESTIMATION

MLR

The MLR can be recorded by frequency-specific brief tones, which have relatively gradual onsets and reasonably long durations. In these stimuli,

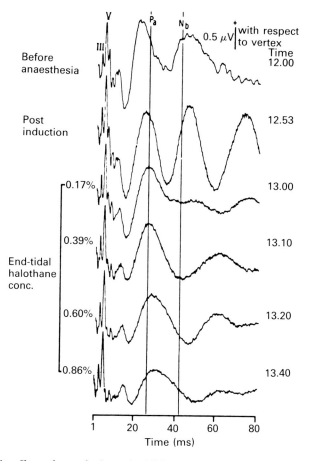

Fig. 8.3 The effects of anaesthesia on the MLR. The latency increases and the amplitude decreases as the halothane concentration increases. The auditory stimulus was a rarefaction click with a dominant frequency of 1 kHz delivered binaurally at 75 dBnHL. (Reproduced with permission from Thornton C et al 1984.)

the energy concentrates at a nominal frequency of the brief tone, and the spread of energy is reasonably narrow.

The MLR thresholds in adults are within 10–20 dBnHL of the behavioural threshold (McFarland et al 1977, Musiek & Geurkink 1981). Good responses can be obtained at low frequencies, and at 500 Hz the responses can be traced to about 10 dBnHL (Kavanagh et al 1984).

The general feeling is that, to clicks and tone pips, the 40 Hz MLR gives better threshold estimation than does MLR at 500, 1000, 2000, and 4000 Hz in both normal adults and in patients with sensorineural hearing loss (Kileny & Shea 1986, Lenarz et al 1986). However, further validation of MLR is required in cases of hearing loss.

Peak amplitudes in infants are smaller than in adults and therefore more difficult to identify at the threshold, and responses to low frequencies are clearer than to high frequency tone bursts. The MLR threshold to clicks in infants aged 12–17 months is at about 40 dBnHL, which is worse than in adults (Horiuchi 1976). For low frequency 500 Hz tone bursts, the MLR thresholds in neonates are similar to those of adults, but at high frequencies the thresholds increase and at 1000, 2000, and 4000 Hz, the thresholds are between 30 and 50 dBnHL (Mendel et al 1977, Frye-Osier et al 1982).

PAM response

The PAM responses sometimes can be used for threshold estimation. Thornton (1975) showed that, if it is recordable, the PAM response is a reasonable threshold estimator, having a response threshold which is approximately 9 dB greater than the subjective audiometric threshold. The standard deviation in differences between subjective and PAM threshold estimates is only 7 dB. Thus, although the response amplitudes vary greatly both within and among subjects, the point at which the response disappears can, nevertheless, provide a good threshold estimate. Again it should be stressed that the absence of a response can give no useful clinical information, as this vestigial, myogenic response is not present in all normal subjects.

MLR IN HEARING AND CNS DISORDERS

For threshold estimation in conductive and cochlear hearing loss, the results for MLR are analogous to those previously described for ECochG and ABR.

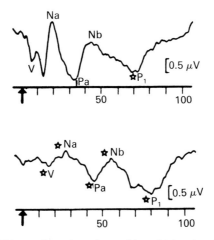

Fig. 8.4 Abnormal MLR waveforms in patients with multiple sclerosis. The indicated components are distorted, and the latencies prolonged. (Reproduced with permission from Rudge P 1983.)

In general, the characteristics of the MLR in peripheral hearing loss are similar to those in normal subjects (McFarland et al 1977).

In brainstem disorders, distortion of the waveform and attenuated or absent Na, Pa, and Nb components were reported in well localized lesions in the brainstem (Yokoyama et al 1987). The amplitudes of the MLR components are very variable, so that the measurement of the latencies is normally used to detect the abnormality. For example, abnormal MLR latencies were found in a considerable number of patients with brainstem tumours and in MS (Rudge 1983). Examples of abnormal MLR in patients with MS are shown in Figure 8.4.

9. The slow vertex response (SVR)

INTRODUCTION

The slow vertex response (SVR), or V potential, arises from the cortical structures. Its main clinical application is in threshold estimation. It is also useful in medicolegal practice to confirm subjective threshold levels, and it has application in assessing hearing in situations of malingering and non-organic hearing loss in adults and adolescents. If passive co-operation can be obtained, the test can be successfully used for those patients with mental handicap or cerebral palsy who cannot give reliable audiometric responses.

GENERATORS OF SLOW-LATENCY RESPONSES

The SVR latency ranges from 50 to 250 ms. The potentials are distributed over the frontal cortex, and they became known as the 'vertex potential' because they were best recorded from the scalp at the vertex (Davis & Zerlin 1966). Topographical studies have shown that contralateral stimulation produces potentials of a larger amplitude than does ipsilateral stimuli (Wolpaw & Penry 1977).

The anatomical and physiologic origins of the SVR are not known, and various waves have several sources. It is thought that SVR is generated in the cerebral cortex, but it is not a primary response because of its latency (Davis 1976). Knight et al (1980) have studied the effects of cortical lesions in man. They have found that frontal lesions do not affect N1 or P2 components; however, extensive temporo-parietal lesions eliminate N1, but not P2.

METHODS

Testing environment

In cortical evoked-response audiometry, the patient is tested with eyes open in order to reduce EEG alpha activity, which may interfere with SVR recording. EEG theta activity can be prominent in some children and also cause problems in SVR recording. Reading is tolerable, but gross body movement, especially muscle activity of the scalp, jaw, and neck, should be avoided, because this causes gross bio-electrical artefacts in ongoing EEG. The patient should be relaxed, reclining in a chair or in a supine position.

Electrode placement

Non-polarizing silver/silver chloride electrodes are used. A pair of active electrodes are placed on the vertex Cz and the peri-auricular region on the mastoid or the auricle M (A). The earth electrode is placed at Fz or on the contralateral peri-auricular region.

Technical aspects of stimulation and recording

Threshold estimation with SVR is similar to that done with a conventional audiometric technique. Usually tone bursts at standard audiometric frequencies are used. The rise and fall times of the tone bursts should be reasonably brief: 10–25 ms with plateaux of about 50–100 ms. There is little evidence that SVR threshold depends significantly on small variations in the duration of the stimuli. The response does not depend on the initial phase of a prolonged tone burst.

The repetition rate should not exceed 1–2/s, in order to avoid adaptation of the response. The number of sweeps per average ranges from 20 to 50, and very rarely up to 128 sweeps may be required in order to obtain good responses. At least two averages should be recorded near threshold and superimposed for greater confidence in identification of the response.

The use of masking noise in the contralateral ear follows normal audiometric rules.

The recommended bandwidth of the filters in the recording amplifiers is 1–30 Hz, and an analysis window of 1/2–1s is used, although in testing children, a longer window is sometimes needed.

NORMATIVE CHARACTERISTICS OF THE SVR

Waveform

Criteria for identification of the response are based on detection of the P1–N1–P2 complex or, at lower stimulus levels, of the N1–P2 peaks (Fig. 9.1).

The SVR consists of several components: P1, N1, P2, and N2. The early P1 component is usually small in adults, and is sometimes difficult to identify. Reduced P1 potential is due to the relatively narrow band-pass filter used. The P1 potential corresponds to the Pb component in the MLR which is better recorded with broader band-pass filters. The N1 component is the most prominent is adults.

In children, the latency and amplitude variation is considerable and can cause some difficulty in interpretation of the components.

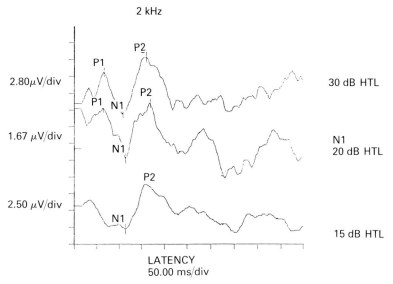

Fig. 9.1   SVRs recorded at 30, 20, and 15 dBnHL.

Amplitude

The N1 and P2 components have the biggest amplitudes, and form the most conspicuous feature of the response. The amplitudes vary from 5 to 15 μV.

Latencies

There is a considerable variation in the latencies of the components of SVR. The early positive wave P1 has a latency of about 50–80 ms; N1, 90–150 ms; P2, 175–250 ms; and N2, 175–300 ms.

Amplitude–intensity and latency–intensity functions

Gradually decreasing the intensity of the stimulus reduces the amplitude and increases the latency of the response. Figure 9.2 shows the N1–P2 potential as a function of stimulus intensity. The amplitude decreases markedly below 50 dBnHL, and the latency is considerably prolonged for stimulus intensities below 30 dBnHL. The latencies near the threshold increase by 50–100%.

FACTORS INFLUENCING CHARACTERISTICS OF NORMAL SVR

Developmental characteristics

In very young children, the immature brain generates large slow potentials on the EEG which may interfere with the response. At term, P2 and N2

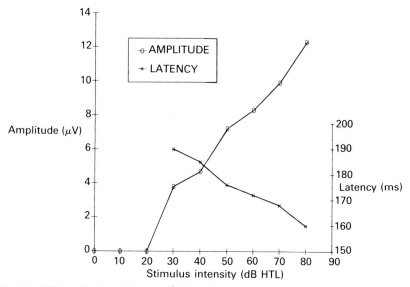

Fig. 9.2 SVR amplitude and latency I/O functions.

can be recognized, and the complete set of major peaks occur in 50–80% of cases when recorded in wakefulness and transient sleep (Rotteveel et al 1986). The adult waveform is reached by the age of 4 months (Engel 1969).

In co-operative older children, the variations in amplitude and latency can cause some difficulty in interpretation.

Sedatives and anaesthetics

Subject attention results in increase of the amplitude of N1 components (Hilliard Picton 1979). However, co-operation and muscle relaxation are very desirable for cortical evoked-response audiometry, especially when SVR applied in difficult-to-test children.

General inhalation anaesthesia and intravenous anaesthesia using thiopentone eliminate SVR and are therefore unsuitable for this purpose.

SVR can be recorded with sedation; however, sedatives modify SVR and impose limitations on its reliability for threshold assessment. In many cases of difficult-to-test children, adequate sedation and sleep are not achieved when using, for example, benzodiazepines, phenothiazines, or barbiturates, and conditions for cortical evoked-response audiometry are unsatisfactory (Hutton 1981).

Phenobarbital sodium has been administered orally or in suppository form, to normal, brain-damaged and deaf infants, in doses of 5–8 mg/kg of body weight (Rapin & Graziani 1967, Burian & Gestring 1971). Changes in the amplitude and latency and small changes in the thresholds of the response have been noticed.

Phenothiazines such as chlorpromazine, in doses 1 mg/kg body weight (Rapin & Graziani 1967) and promethazine 1 mg/kg body weight (Beagley et al 1972, Karnahl & Benning 1972), were reported as giving satisfactory testing conditions for SVR, and produced less change in response than did benzodiazepine (diazepam) and barbiturates.

FREQUENCY SPECIFICITY OF SVR AND THRESHOLD ESTIMATION

Using long tone bursts, one can construct an audiogram, and the SVR can be used to estimate hearing threshold on low and high audiometric frequencies to within 10 dB in almost all patients (Hyde et al 1986).

SVR IN HEARING AND CNS DISORDERS

In conductive and cochlear hearing loss, the thresholds for SVR correspond to the behavioural thresholds and are within 20 dBnHL (Davies et al 1967, Beagley & Kellogg 1969).

Bone-conduction audiograms can resolve air-bone gaps in conductive hearing loss; however, the procedure is lengthy.

In CNS disorders, the SVR is not a sensitive indicator of lesions. However, abnormalities of the SVR depend on the extent of the lesion. Abnormal SVR was reported by Rudge (1983) in a case of cortical deafness. The temporo-parietal lesions cause marked reduction on N1, but not P2 (Knight et al 1982). Abnormal N1–P2 components with extensive temporo-parietal infarcts were reported by Mauguière et al (1982).

10. Other long latency responses

Of these other responses, the one that is most useful in the auditory field is the vertex positive component P3 or P300 with a latency of about 300 ms (see Fig. 2.7). The P3 potential is thought to be associated with a number of cognitive processes and with the short-term memory function (Goodin et al 1978, Hillyard 1984). The scalp topography of the P3 amplitude is maximal in the central-parietal mid-line area, and it is bilaterally symmetric (Simson et al 1977). After measuring intracranial potentials, Halgren et al (1980) suggested that P3 is an endogenous potential generated in subcortical structures such as the hippocampal formation and the amygdala. Goff et al (1980), using intracranial recordings, suggested that neural origins of late-latency evoked potentials may be associated with deep-brain structures, and may not be directly generated from the cortical surface.

There are also slow direct-current potentials of cortical origin associated with expectancy; these are described by Walter (1964) as contingent negative variation (CNV), which is a pre-signal potential; it is schematically shown in Figure 2.5.

METHODS

The P300 can be readily observed as a component of the auditory event-related potential (see Fig. 2.7) in an 'oddball' paradigm. This paradigm requires the processing of task-relevant information, in which the subject detects and, for example, counts 'target' tones that occur randomly in a sequence of 'non-target' tones (Sutton et al 1965). About 20–30 replications may suffice to record it. The filter characteristics are similar to those used in recording SVR.

CLINICAL APPLICATIONS

Several studies have used the P300 component to investigate normal and disordered cognitive processes (Fig. 10.1) (Goodin 1978, Hillyard 1984, Sklare & Lynn 1984). No effect on P300 amplitude was present when the

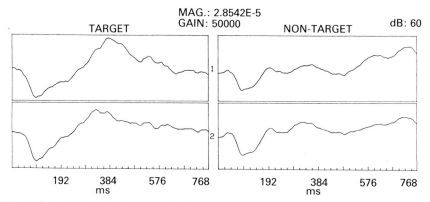

Fig. 10.1A P300 results in a normal subject. 'Target tones' of 100 ms duration at 1500 Hz were delivered 30% of the time (30 targets). The 'non-target tones' of 100 ms duration at 1000 Hz were delivered 70% of the time (70 non-target). Stimulus level is 60 dB. Recordings FzM (top) and CzM (bottom).

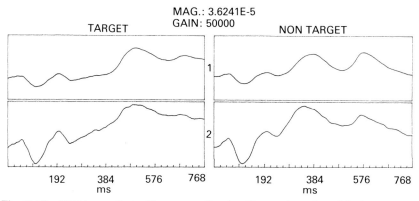

Fig. 10.1B P300 in a patient with memory disorder. Note prolongation of the latency. (With permission of Prasher D, The National Hospitals for Nervous Diseases, London.)

stimulus intensity was increased, but there was a decrease in the latency (Papanicolaou et al 1985). The latency of P300 increases regularly with increasing age from 20 to 79 years, at a rate of 1.3 ms/year, but its amplitude decreases (Picton et al 1984). Prolonged latency of P300 was found in some patients with dementia (Gordon et al 1986).

Whilst the CNV has potential application to disorders of the higher brain, it has not been possible to realize a technique for routine clinical application.

Electric response audiometry testing strategies

11. Comparative assessment of ERA threshold techniques

In order to apply the numerous ERA techniques appropriately, it is important to know their comparative merits in particular clinical situations. The clinical factors include, for example, how evoked-response threshold techniques may be affected by the age and state of the patient, the need for general anaesthesia, the possible site of the lesion, and the accuracy needed for practical purposes.

IDENTIFICATION OF THE RESPONSE

The technical and interpretive expertise required for ERA tests is greater than for conventional audiometry. Although they are objective tests, the judgement of the presence of the response and measurement of the diagnostic parameters are subjective. Technical experience is essential, especially as some of the tests are more difficult than others, and failure to recognize the responses may lead to inadequate evaluation of the results.

Automatic response recognition is desirable and is possible within certain limitations, but, ultimately, there is currently no substitute for an experienced tester. Furthermore, poor-quality recording is unlikely to be compensated for by automatic signal processing.

Auditory-evoked potentials are the averages from ongoing bio-electrical activity and ambient electrical noise. The signal-to-noise ratio is one of the most important factors for good-quality recordings, and it is up to the tester to decide the intensity of the stimuli, number of sweeps, number of replications, artefact rejection limits, and other technical recording factors, although some laboratory systems continue averaging until a certain S/N ratio is attained. Both physiologic and non-physiologic electrical noise can have an effect on test duration, threshold sensitivity, and threshold variability. Nevertheless, even in non-ideal conditions, an adequate response may be obtained (Fig. 11.1).

Passive co-operation by the patient is adequate for most non-invasive ERA tests. However, natural sleep in babies, sedation, or general anaesthesia may be required to keep the patient still and reduce excessive myogenic activity. In many anxious patients, an oral dose of diazepam reduces muscle activity in the scalp, around the jaws, and in the neck.

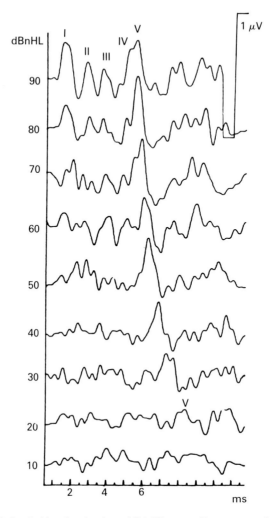

Fig. 11.1 ABR threshold estimation in a child. The recordings were made in an electrically unscreened operating theatre. Whilst the traces are 'noisy', the prominent wave V can, nevertheless, be detected and the threshold estimate made.

Electrical interference can considerably reduce the quality of the recording. It may be a problem when the tests are carried out in neonatal units or operating theatres. All non-essential electrical equipment, especially fluorescent lights, should be switched off.

Transtympanic electrocochleography has the best signal-to-noise ratio of the early responses, and detection and interpretation are comparatively easier than in other evoked potentials. Transtympanic ECochG can be carried out with only local anaesthesia in a co-operative adult, but in a child it requires general anaesthesia. Fortunately, sedation and general anaesthesia do not degrade the response.

Interpretation of the SVR may be more difficult, as there may be myogenic artefacts, as well as contamination by prominent alpha and theta rhythmical activity on the EEG. The subject's eyes should be open in order to reduce alpha rhythm. The SVR is known to be a stimulus-orientated response, and is usually recorded easily in a patient who anticipates the stimulus. Natural sleep and general anaesthesia have an effect on both EEG and SVR, making identification of the response at the threshold more difficult.

Interpretative skills for MLR in conscious co-operative patients are similar to those needed for SVR. The response is also affected by general anaesthesia. A clearer response can be achieved by stimulating at a rate of 40 stimuli/s, which is called the 40 Hz MLR response.

At present, ABR is used more often than other ERA tests in infants and in neuro-otologic patients. ABR is not affected by sedation or general anaesthesia, and myogenic activity can thus be reduced to improve the quality of the recording. Accurate measurement of the latencies of the peaks of the response is required for neuro-otologic testing, and the latencies should be compared with normative data, using similar stimulation and recording parameters.

Myogenic auditory-evoked potentials, such as the postauricular muscle response (PAM), vary with the state of muscular tonus at a particular time, and, therefore, are less suitable for audiometric assessment than neurogenic auditory-evoked potentials.

CLINICAL CONSIDERATIONS OF THE PROCEDURE

ECochG requires the placement of the electrode by an otologist through the tympanic membrane. In any patient (i.e. children, the mentally handicapped, etc.) who is incapable of lying still or who cannot be trusted to avoid turning onto the electrode, general anaesthesia is required.

For all other test situations, ERA can be performed by the technical staff in conscious patients. A relaxed state is required for all tests except the PAM, and there must be minimal body movement, scalp or neck muscle movement, and jaw clenching. The best recordings are obtained in relaxed patients in a supine position. Eye closure, natural sleep, and general anaesthesia improve recordings of ABR, but may have an adverse effect on the detection of SVR, which is thought to be of cortical origin. Therefore, for SVR, the patient should be awake with his eyes open.

If the patient is hyperactive and not testable with SVR because of gross myogenic electrical artefacts, it is unlikely that good responses will be obtained by trying to record ABR or MLR in similar conditions, although PAM recording may be successful.

Natural sleep after a feed is an ideal condition for testing neonates with ABR and MLR. In older infants, sedation may be required, which can be administered orally or per rectum. For children who are difficult to test, including those that are hyperactive or have brain damage, mental handicap, or behavioural problems, sedation may not be adequate, and they may need light general anaesthesia in order to achieve good recording conditions. It is unnecessary to use muscle relaxants, although they can improve the recordings further. Some clinics have reported that transtympanic ECochG in adults may cause momentary discomfort when placing the electrode, but most patients tolerate transtympanic needle ECochG well, even without local anaesthesia. Local anaesthetic sprays and iontophoresis have been used to anaesthetize the tympanic membrane, but their effectiveness is variable.

The duration of testing, especially for threshold assessment, is an important factor in the clinical application of auditory-evoked potentials. ECochG using broad-band clicks requires the least testing time. Click-evoked ABR requires more time than does ECochG, but the testing time can be reduced by increasing the stimulation rate to 30/s or more, without compromising threshold estimation. However, the waveform of the response may be affected. For example, the screening time for the threshold using click-evoked ABR in a sleeping neonate typically takes about 20 minutes. Frequency-specific responses from ECochG and ABR can be obtained, but it is a very time-consuming procedure and may not be practical in every circumstance. A frequency-specific air-conduction SVR audiogram, at four frequencies in both ears, in an adult or adolescent can be completed in about an hour. The 40 Hz MLR compares similarly in testing time with SVR; however, there has been less validation in cases of hearing loss.

The risks associated with ERA should be considered. Complications may occur if general anaesthesia is used, and those compromising the laryngeal airway in children are serious. (Crowley et al 1976) reported that 3 out of 603 patients known to have had general anaesthesia experienced laryngospasm. ECochG results from different centres have been assessed in 2256 patients, of whom 13 who had local or general anaesthesia experienced nausea, vomiting, and vertigo. Acute otitis media was reported in 2 out of 1875 patients following transtympanic ECochG, which is a risk of about 0.1% (Crowley et al 1976). Out of more than 3000 transtympanic ECochG reported by Gibson et al (1983), 1 patient complained that his trigeminal neuralgia was worse for 2 months following the test, and another patient complained that his tinnitus had become louder.

FREQUENCY SPECIFICITY OF ERA TESTS

Estimation of the audiogram with ERA involves a consideration of factors such as the acoustic properties of the brief stimuli, the spread of excitation along the basilar membrane, and electrophysiologic tuning of the primary neurones in impaired cochleae. The early evoked potentials, CAP and ABR, require good neural synchrony and, hence, use fast onset short-duration stimuli. The shorter the stimulus duration, the greater the spread of energy over frequency. Broad-band clicks excite practically the whole cochlea, and very brief tones also have a wide spread of energy. Therefore, brief tones are not ideal as frequency-specific stimuli.

The later evoked potentials, such as MLR and especially SVR, can be recorded by more frequency-specific stimuli, which have relatively gradual onset and reasonably long duration. The spread of energy of these stimuli is considerably less.

The good synchronization of early evoked potentials is achieved by excitation of the basal part of the cochlea. As the travelling wave progresses towards the apical turn, the synchrony for lower frequencies diminishes, and out-of-phase single-fibre responses contribute little to the compound response. Thus, the CAP represents mainly electrophysiologic activity in the basal turn of the cochlea and gives little information about frequencies lower than 2000 Hz. For all early evoked potentials, the problem of acoustic energy spread and excitation spread along the basilar membrane limits the frequency specificity of the responses. However, the representation of lower frequencies in ABR, as reflected in wave V, is greater than in the CAP. Neither ECochG nor ABR audiometry with brief tone bursts guarantee adequate frequency specificity. A further factor should be considered, namely that in cochlear lesions the tuning mechanism and frequency specificity of single neurones may be affected.

In order to obtain better frequency-specific responses, it is possible to alter cochlear responsiveness by masking with ipsilateral noise the parts of the cochlea which are not stimulated with tone bursts. High-pass noise masking and derived response techniques can be used. Alternatively, more complicated band-pass masking with noise or notched-noise masking can be used.

THRESHOLD ESTIMATION

The difference between ERA and the behavioural estimates of threshold in normal subjects produces a 'correction' factor for clinical use. In practice, the correction factor's value does not matter, provided that it is sufficiently small to obviate problems due to recruitment or to the limits of the audiometer's maximum stimulus intensity. For example, if the correction factor is 50 dB, then to measure the evoked response threshold for a patient with a 70 dB loss, would require stimulation levels greater than 120 dB. Clearly, if there is a recruiting loss, such a large correction factor will lead to inaccurate estimates.

Good experience and skill in all techniques is a prerequisite for the comparative assessment of the techniques. Because so many factors may affect accurate measurement of ERA, each laboratory should establish its own data, emulating those published, as a guideline.

A lesion of the auditory pathway can have an effect upon detection of the auditory evoked potentials. The presence of neural dysfunction caused by disruption of neural synchrony may not reveal a hearing loss on a pure-tone audiogram. However, ABR can be totally eliminated by the effects, for example, of multiple sclerosis in the brainstem, or a small acoustic tumour. On rare occasions, the absence of the response is idiopathic. The MLR and

SVR are less dependent on neuronal synchrony, and less sensitive to the effect of a lesion, allowing threshold estimates which can be largely independent of disorders creating neural asynchrony, in the same way as a subjective pure-tone audiogram. Peripheral lesions, causing hearing loss on the audiogram, will be reflected by most ERA tests. However, a lesion more rostral than the site of the generator of the evoked potential may give a normal estimate of the threshold in the presence of hearing loss. For example, a normal CAP can be recorded in a patient with a brainstem lesion due to multiple sclerosis; or a normal ABR and MLR can be recorded in a patient with cortical deafness (Ozdamar et al 1982).

Assuming equally good test conditions, one can use the following threshold correction factors as a guideline. The SVR sensitivity is about 5 dB at audiometric frequencies 500–4000 Hz. As it has good frequency specificity, the SVR can resolve any audiometric contour, including notched hearing loss. The 40-Hz MLR correction factor is close to that of the SVR; however, further validation in cases of hearing loss is required. The ABR elicited by clicks has a correction factor of about 15 dB in a flat or gradually sloping audiogram. The ABR in response to frequency-specific stimuli has a correction factor of about 20 dB at frequencies 1000–4000 Hz. For lower frequencies, ABR has limitations, and the correction factor increases to about 30 dB. The ABR using tone-burst stimuli has a similarly high correction factor and is thus limited in estimating severe hearing loss. With transtympanic ECochG, the signal-to-noise ratio is good, and the AP has a sensitivity to clicks and tone bursts at frequencies of 2000 Hz and higher of about 10 dB or less. At lower frequencies, the sensitivity of ECochG decreases considerably. Clinical experience indicates that the better S/N ratio occurring with ECochG enables it to estimate severe high frequency hearing loss better than ABR. The correction factor of ECochG and ABR depends on the audiometric contour, and it is better for flat audiograms than for high frequency, steeply sloping ones.

As a result of many acoustic, electrophysiologic, and recording factors, no single ERA test is best for all applications, and the test should be chosen bearing in mind the above mentioned factors. Sometimes a combination of ERA tests has to be considered in order to achieve a diagnosis.

For example, if responses from more peripheral generators indicate a low or near normal threshold, whilst those from more rostral generators indicate a greater hearing loss, in agreement with a subjective audiogram, then the site of the disorder may be estimated to lie between the most rostral generator, which gives a 'low' threshold estimate, and the most peripheral generator, which gives a 'high' threshold estimate. Note that, in general, CNS lesions, unless they are bilateral or very large, do not cause an audiometric hearing loss.

In particular, a normal or near normal threshold estimate from wave I (ECochG) for a unilateral loss is an excellent indicator of a medially located VIIIth nerve lesion.

CONCLUSIONS ABOUT FEATURES OF ERA TESTS

Some general audiometric features of various ERA tests are summarized in Table 11.1.

Table 11.1   ERA audiometric features in estimating hearing loss

Feature	ECochG	ABR	PAM	MLR	SVR
Value as a threshold estimator (2–4 kHz)	good	good	poor	good	good
Threshold correction factor (2–4 kHz)	0–5 dB	10–20 dB	10–20 dB (absence inconclusive)	10–20 dB	0–10 dB
Frequency specificity (for tone-burst stimuli)	poor	poor	bad	good	very good
Threshold dependency on brainstem lesion	no	yes	yes	yes	no
Effect of sleep/sedation/ gen. anaesthesia	no	no	yes (on muscle tonus)	yes	yes

The positive features of the SVR include its generation from the cortical structures, its good threshold sensitivity and good frequency specificity, and its relative insensitivity to CNS lesions. These features make SVR a good audiometric tool, with particular value for estimating thresholds both in functional hearing loss in adults and in medicolegal cases. However, the disadvantages of SVR are that it is affected by sleep, sedation, and general anaesthesia, and is therefore not applicable to babies and difficult-to-test children.

MLR is thought to be generated in the thalamus, and to have good frequency specificity. However, its threshold sensitivity and variability in the presence of hearing loss have not been sufficiently evaluated.

As for myogenic middle-latency responses, of which PAM is the most commonly known, these are not always present in normal subjects, and depend on the tonus of the muscles. Whilst middle latency responses can give good threshold estimates if a response is present, they are not, in general, a good method of audiometric assessment, particularly in young children, in whom the tonus may change suddenly, for example, in sleep.

ABR is very useful both in neuro-otological diagnosis and in threshold estimation by wave V detection. ABR is a very stable response, and its variability both within and among subjects is small, which makes its latencies suitable as diagnostic parameters. ABR is not significantly affected by sleep, sedation, and general anaesthesia, making it a good tool for estimating behavioural hearing levels in babies and children who are difficult to test. The threshold sensitivity for clicks is good in the region of 2000–4000 Hz. However, the detailed audiometric contour does not correlate well with tone-burst evoked ABR; notched hearing loss and low and high frequency loss may not be estimated unless ipsilateral noise masking of the appropriate parts of the cochlea is applied.

As for transtympanic ECochG, it has very good threshold sensitivity in response to clicks and tone pips at audiometric frequencies at and above 2000 Hz. However, its frequency specificity has the same limitations as that of ABR, and it is poor for frequencies below 1000 Hz, though adequate at higher frequencies. The main disadvantage of ECochG is that it is invasive and requires general anaesthesia for children. It also requires the expertise of the otologist as opposed to that of the audiometric technician, in order to place the ECochG electrode. Hence, CAP reflects peripheral changes at the level of the cochlea, and, together with ABR, it can be a helpful test in neuro-otological diagnosis.

12. ERA in hearing screening in neonates and infants

CLINICAL PROBLEM

There is general agreement about the desirability of early detection and management of hearing loss. Even a comparatively mild hearing impairment can cause considerable speech abnormality and may delay the development of communication skills.

Various hearing screening programmes have been suggested, raising the questions of the selection of population to be screened, which tests to use, and what level of hearing loss one should aim to identify.

Population

Accurate hearing levels are difficult to measure in early infancy, and the epidemiological picture is inadequate. A World Health Organization (WHO) report (1967) suggests that the incidence of severe hearing loss in neonates is about 1:1000, and that of some degree of hearing impairment may be as high as 5:1000.

Certain children have an increased risk of hearing loss and are in a special 'at risk' group. It has been shown that in some groups, for example, very low birth-weight children (less than 1500 g) in intensive care, the incidence of bilateral severe hearing loss is 4% and the incidence of any degree of hearing loss, including mild and unilateral, reaches 9% for those aged 3–6 years (Abramovich et al 1979). It should be noted that low birth-weight alone is not a 'risk' factor for hearing loss. However, factors such as perinatal illness, particularly those conditions, including apnoea, known or likely to have caused hypoxia in the neonatal period, are significantly associated with sensorineural hearing loss, and jaundice appears to have an additive effect (Abramovich et al 1979). A register of the main risk factors is a useful way of identifying children who are most likely to suffer impaired hearing and who, therefore, need reliable testing. A practical version of a risk register, similar to that proposed by the Joint Committee on Infant Hearing (1982), has proved useful; it includes the following factors:

1. Family history of childhood hearing impairment
2. Congenital perinatal infections

3. Anatomical malformations involving head and neck
4. Birth-weight less than 1500 g
5. Hyperbilirubinaemia
6. Asphyxia with acidosis

The Joint Committee on Infant Hearing (1982) has estimated the incidence of moderate to profound hearing loss at 2.5–5% in the 'at risk' group. The incidence of risk factors is under 5%, and, as most babies with risk factors 1 and 3 (above) are to be found in the normal wards, the high-risk group is not necessarily concentrated among those infants treated in special-care baby units. In these groups, the incidence of severe hearing loss increases by at least tenfold, and that of some degree of hearing loss increases by much more. Some risk factors, for example, recessive familial hearing loss, viral infections and asphyxia depend on the investigation pattern for detection, and are especially prone to variability. About 95% of babies do not fall into a risk category; however, one should bear in mind that only half of the children with a hearing loss manifest a known risk factor (Simmons 1980, Feinmesser et al 1982, Stein et al 1983). This emphasizes the need for general awareness of the possibility of hearing loss.

It is relatively easy to schedule children from the special baby-care units; however, it is unsatisfactory to restrict testing to only this group of children. Systematic assessment of risk factors in the general nursery would be a major undertaking. Therefore, it is imperative that all medical practitioners involved in paediatrics become familiar with the risk categories and refer such children for early testing.

CHOICE OF SCREENING TESTS

Both behavioural and non-invasive electrophysiologic tests have been suggested and tried in early hearing loss detection. Various screening programmes have been suggested to assess the hearing of babies just before they leave hospital, or at a later date within the first 6 months of life.

The value of a test depends on its sensitivity and specificity. The sensitivity is the probability of a positive screen, which signifies the presence of a hearing loss. The specificity is the probability of a negative screen. A negative screen means that the test shows hearing within normal limits. It is important to avoid false-negative error rates, because this means missing identification of a hearing loss. False-positive error rates are undesirable, because they cause a false alarm which may lead to parental anxiety and further unnecessary investigations. Of two tests with the same sensitivity, the test which has a higher specificity is more valuable. However, one should bear in mind that the clinician's skill and experience influence the error rate of any technique.

Observational audiometry and automated behavioural screening tests, such as the auditory-response cradle, identify neonates with severe and profound hearing loss fairly reliably (Feinmesser & Tell 1976, Bennett 1979, 1980, Weiss 1983, Bhattacharya et al 1984). Several reports have indicated high error rates with the standard behavioural tests and with the automated auditory-response cradle (Feinmesser & Tell 1976, Northern & Downs 1978, Davies 1984, McCormick et al 1984).

Oto-acoustic emissions from the cochlea recorded by means of a very sensitive microphone in the ear canal, are being evaluated as a screening test in neonates, and the initial data appear to reflect the results obtained in adults, namely that for hearing losses of greater than 30 dB HTL, the evoked emission is absent. It is a particularly suitable technique for neonatal screening, as neonates have a much larger evoked emission than do adults.

Auditory-evoked potentials have been used with enthusiasm by many investigators. ECochG is undesirable because it is an invasive procedure requiring general anaesthesia. The ABR, easily recorded in sleeping neonates and infants, seems to be superior to other tests in the screening of mild to profound hearing loss using broad-band clicks (Fig. 12.1, A, B, C). Frequency specificity can be improved by masking parts of the cochlea with band-stop or high-pass masking noise.

The postauricular muscle response (PAM) has been used for screening neonates and infants (Douek et al 1973, Fraser et al 1978). PAM depends on the tonus of the scalp muscles and is elicited only at relatively high intensities. It gives a high false-positive error rate, which limits its usefulness.

The middle-latency responses (MLR) and 40 Hz MLR have limited application in neonatal hearing screening. It has been reported that the MLR may be difficult to recognize in a sleeping neonate, and is less consistent and more difficult to record than ABR (Ozdamar & Kraus 1983, Rotteveel et al 1986). Frye-Osier & Hirsch (1980) tested normal neonates and recorded MLRs in response to 500; 2000; and 4000 Hz tone bursts at levels of 10, 30, and 50 dBnHL. The MLR was recordable at the 10 dB level for the 500 Hz stimulus and at the 30 dB level for the 4000 Hz stimulus, but only at the 50 dB level for the 2000 Hz stimulus. There is clear evidence of maturational changes in the MLR as it is symmetrically distributed over the scalp in adults, but show marked asymmetry in neonates (Wolf & Goldstein 1978). Both the MLR and the 40 Hz MLR thresholds are reported to increase in the sleeping infant. However, both the MLR and the 40 Hz MLR are more frequency-specific than ABR when using tone pips, and can be of value to assess hearing in the low frequencies. The middle-latency responses, including MLR, 40 Hz MLR, and SN10 can be considered in some difficult cases to supplement hearing investigation in a test battery.

The SVR is frequency specific, but in a sleeping infant the waveforms are unpredictable and variable.

In conclusion, ABR is the test of choice for screening neonates and infants with broad-band frequency clicks. If a more detailed audiometric contour

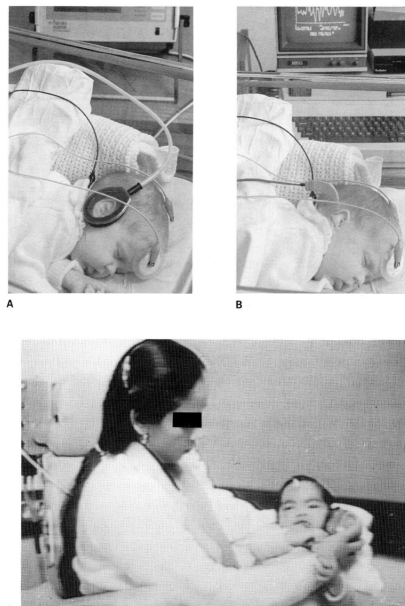

Fig. 12.1 (**A**) The Algotek screener in use on a neonate. Acoustic stimuli are delivered by plastic tubes to a circumaural, sealed cavity. This avoids the closure of the ear canal, which can occur with earphones. (**B**) ABR responses being recorded from a neonate. A miniature insert transducer is used to deliver the stimulus. (**C**) ABR screening of a 4-month-old child. The mother holds the earphone a few centimetres from the ear.

is required, then some frequency specificity can be achieved by masking with the techniques of band-stop or high-pass masking noise. Other more frequency-specific MLR potentials can be recorded to assess hearing loss at low audiometric frequencies. Available ERA tests for screening along with the recommended parameters are shown in Table 12.1.

Table 12.1 ERA tests for screening

Test	ABR	PAM	MLR
Stimulus	click ±	click ±	click ± (tone burst; see text)
Rate	20–40/s	10–20/s	5–10/s
Number of averages	2048	300	256–512
Level	30–40 dBnHL 60–70 dBnHL	50 dBnHL	50 dBnHL (500 Hz; see text)
Filter pass-band	40–3000 Hz	100–3000 Hz	30–300 Hz

SCREENING WITH ABR

Using ABR, one can design the screening programme to detect any degree of hearing loss, including mild, moderate, and unilateral. For this purpose, low testing levels of 30–40 dBnHL are used. When the aim is to screen for moderate to moderate-severe hearing loss, a higher stimulus level of 60–70 dBnHL has been recommended. Auditory threshold measurement is based on wave V, since it can be detected to within 15 dB of the behavioural threshold.

Screening neonates by means of ABR was first proposed by Galambos (1978). Screening just before discharge from hospital sometimes results in a non-ideal test environment, such as in a quiet office adjoining the nursery. Of 368 babies screened in the room adjoining the nursery, where the steady noise level was 55 dBA, only 63% passed at 30 dBnHL (Abramovich et al 1987). However, after increasing stimulus intensity by 10 dB to 40 dBnHL, the pass rate reached 84%, reducing unilateral and bilateral failures by more than half, or by, respectively, 11 and 5% (Table 12.2).

Predischarge screening with clicks in an environment, better controlled audiometrically, as in the sound-proof room, shows that many babies who failed the screen at 30 dB in the nursery gave clear responses in the audiometrically better environment within 24 hours. Comparing predischarge-screening results (with moderate click intensities) in the nursery with the results in the sound-proof room, it appears that the failure rate halves in an audiometrically better environment. The test was done on 250 babies who were drawn equally from the special baby-care unit and the general nursery. There was considerable improvement of the test outcome; 82% of babies passed at 30 dBnHL, and 92% at 40 dBnHL, including 6%

Table 12.2   Screening with click-evoked ABR

		Predischarge ABR in nursery room (%)	Predischarge ABR in audiometric room (%)	At 3 months, ABR in audiometric room (%)
30 dBnHL	Pass	63	82	89
	Fail			
	unilat.	24	12	5
	bilat.	13	6	6
40 dBnHL	Pass	84	92	95
	Fail			
	unilat.	11	6	3
	bilat.	5	2	2

of unilateral and 2% of bilateral failures. This suggests that there is a considerable incidence of mild hearing loss in the neonatal period, although developmental factors could contribute to the failure rates.

Environmental effects, such as ambient acoustic and electrical noise, contribute to the considerable failure rates, especially when one tests in the nursery with the hand-held headphones. Noise-excluding circumaural headphone cushions are unlikely to be effective or suitable with neonates, and they may press on the ear, producing ear canal collapse. It appears, therefore, that screening for hearing loss, including mild and moderate loss, in the nursery may yield excessive false-positive failure rates. Between 10 and 20% of high-risk neonates fail an ABR screen in the nursery for a click stimulus at 30–40 dBnHL (Galambos et al 1982, Alberti et al 1983, Sanders et al 1985).

A proportion of infants who fail an initial ABR screening test pass it when retested several months later. This could be due to transient changes in the middle ear or to transient neurological abnormalities in the neonatal period, the latter affecting recording of ABR. Therefore, a follow-up test or initial screening at 3–5 months is recommended. Testing of 466 children at 3–4 months has revealed that there was resolution of hearing loss in some children, although in several a hearing loss emerged. All the cases of developing hearing loss were mild and unilateral. Overall, there was some further improvement in the outcomes, and the pass rate was 89% at 30 dB, and at 40-dBnHL clicks the pass rate was 95% with 2% bilateral and 3% unilateral failures (Abramovich et al 1986).

Stimulation using bone conduction may avoid screening failures due to possible middle-ear disease, but exhibit failures due to sensorineural hearing loss. Stimulation using bone conduction will spread into both ears, and will reflect ABR threshold from the better cochlea. This is desirable for screening purposes for neonates for whom only bilateral losses will require management, but will mean that appropriate masking techniques are needed for diagnosis.

At present, there is no more accurate diagnostic test for very early hearing-loss detection against which to assess the screening performance of ABR for mild, moderate, and unilateral hearing loss. The obtained results should be carefully assessed clinically, and one should refrain from a technical judgement of false-positive or false-negative ABR. According to a 1-year follow-up study, which included questionnaires sent to physicians and parents (Abramovich et al 1987) and behavioural testing (Bradford et al 1985), there was not one case of hearing loss or false-negative ABR results in a child who passed an ABR test at 3–4 months.

Hearing-loss estimation

The correlation between ABR and behavioural thresholds is sufficient to be of great use in the early identification of hearing loss. In the absence of grossly abnormal ABR waveforms, it is assumed, though cautiously, that the test reflects true hearing sensitivity. In general, screening with ABR is a practical and viable procedure for babies who are well and who are over 40 weeks of gestational age.

Good responses can be obtained at 30–40 dBnHL low-intensity click stimuli in an audiometrically adequate environment.

Little is gained by screening for mild hearing loss in the acoustically inadequate environment of the nursery. Environmental effects contribute to poor specificity in the 30-dB screen and would generate a considerable load on follow-up testing. Therefore, 40 dBnHL clicks are favoured in this environment.

The screening test parameters have significant effects on sensitivity and specificity. Since the objective is efficiently to detect wave V of the evoked response, not to make detailed waveform measurement, a relatively high stimulation rate is appropriate, and stimulation rates of 30/s or higher are used.

If a baby fails screening before leaving hospital, a follow-up at 3–4 months is essential. Priority of follow-up is given to those children failing at higher screening levels, for example at a click intensity of 60 dBnHL. The general feeling is that substantial predischarge hearing loss tends to be sustained at the follow-up, whereas there is some resolution of genuine mild hearing loss. However, there has been a reported case of severe hearing loss before discharge, which totally resolved itself at 4 months; the risk factor was severe perinatal asphyxia (Abramovich et al 1987).

Low and high frequency hearing in sleeping infants can be assessed with ABR. It is possible to assess low, middle, and high frequencies with ABR at, say, 500 Hz with a notch-filtered masking-noise method, or by using a high-pass noise masking method (Fig. 12.2). The more frequency-specific slow-vertex response (SVR) is less predictable in a sleeping child.

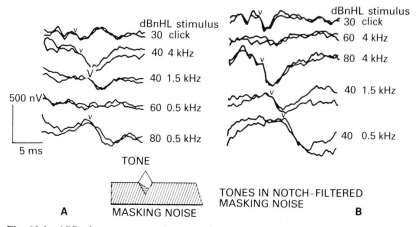

Fig. 12.2 ABRs from neonates using tones in notch-noise. (**A**) A case with a marked, low-frequency loss giving no response at 60 dB to a 500-Hz stimulus. (**B**) A case with a high-frequency loss giving no response at 60 dB to a 4000-Hz stimulus. (After Hyde 1985.)

The audiometric profile was assessed by using 500, 1500, and 4000 Hz tone bursts in notch-filtered (a variation of band-reject filter) noise. About 150 neonates were tested before discharge, and more than 250 infants were tested at follow-ups 3–4 months later. Failure for tone bursts was based on 40 dBnHL stimuli, as it is more difficult, purely on technical grounds, to detect responses to tone bursts at lower intensities. The ABR results of high-frequency, 4000 Hz tone bursts were similar to those for clicks. The failure rate for low frequency, 500 Hz tone pips was considerable in the neonatal period, but 4 months later the failure rates halved (Abramovich et al 1987). Most low frequency hearing deficits were mild and undetected by testing with the clicks. In a small proportion of infants, low frequency hearing deficits emerged. It appears that many low frequency hearing deficits were of middle-ear origin. The results of predischarge and follow-up ABRs show a considerable amount of change during the first trimester of life, especially with regard to mild or low frequency hearing loss. Detailed audiometric contour assessment is feasible at about 4 months of age, especially in those infants who have failed a test using click stimuli. In sleeping infants, the ABR tests can be supplemented with more frequency-specific MLR tests.

Screening ABR strategies

Because of the small percentage of mild neonatal hearing losses that resolve themselves by the age of 3–4 months, predischarge ABR screening should have its failures checked with another test such as evoked acoustic emissions. This helps to determine neurological disease in which the ABR is absent or abnormal, but in which the hearing may be normal.

Predischarge screening, both in the automated-cradle and oto-acoustic emission tests, has been suggested as a determinant of follow-up ABR testing at 3–4 months. Further evaluation of this strategy is required.

Certain risk factors may be associated with progressive impairment, and, therefore, some clinicians prefer to delay the ABR until the infant is 3 months old, that is to say, until some time before the age at which hearing rehabilitation should begin. At this age, results are less influenced by residual neonatal problems or factors relating to the development of the hearing pathway. One should be careful not to present parents with potentially incorrect ABR test results, especially in the neonatal period. We also strongly argue the rationale of follow-up testing at 3 months. In some centres it may be more convenient to schedule babies for ABR testing at 3 months of age. However, in some cases of marked risk factors and predictably low parental compliance in return ABR testing, it is advisable to test the baby before it leaves the hospital.

In general, neonates, particularly if they are tested during sleep following a feed, are easier to test than 3 month old babies, who more often remain awake and active.

Optimal test parameters must be selected in order to make the test quick and efficient. The usual recommendations are given in Table 12.1. The clicks are delivered at recommended intensity levels of 30–40 dBnHL or 60–70 dBnHL through a hand-held TDH-type earphone to each ear separately.

The practicality of testing requires the babies to be asleep. This can be achieved by testing the babies following a scheduled feed, and maternal participation may be required. Once the baby is asleep and the electrodes attached, it takes, typically, about 20 minutes to do an ABR screen with clicks.

The testing procedure starts by presenting the click at 30–40 dBnHL, and if the ABR response is normal, the baby is considered to have passed the test. If the ABR response at 40 dBnHL is absent, the intensity of the click stimulus should be raised to 60–70 dBnHL, and the baby retested. The presence of normal response at 60–70 dBnHL click intensity warrants investigation for mild to moderate hearing loss. Predischarge screening should be followed by a detailed ABR test within the next 3 months, as well as otoscopic examination. Impedance audiometry to detect middle-ear dysfunction is useful, but this method has limitations for those under 6 months of age (Paradise 1982).

If the ABR is absent at 60–70 dBnHL, one should consider the possibility of a severe hearing loss. Neurological status, especially in the very low birthweight babies who may have suffered intracranial haemorrhage or asphyxia, could have a confounding effect on both the threshold and morphology of ABR. These infants should be retested with a broad-band click and at low frequency within 3 months, so that rehabilitation can start early. These thresholds, as well as a neurological ABR assessment, usually can be obtained within 1 hour, given careful parental instructions and correct test methodology. If the baby refuses to sleep, testing can often be done during feeding, giving careful attention to EEG monitoring and myogenic artefact rejection. If the baby wakes up within 30 minutes, and is not testable, then he can be rescheduled for ABR tests. It is important to rule out significant bilateral hearing loss, and it is desirable to test each ear with a click quickly. Neither turning the baby to test the other ear, nor potentially arousing acoustic stimuli are likely to awaken it during a 20 minute period after feeding.

Overall, it appears that ABR is, at present, the most useful audiometric tool for early hearing evaluation and can contribute a great deal to early hearing loss detection and management. When resources are limited, it is sensible to concentrate initially on testing in high-risk groups, although only half of the children with a hearing loss will manifest a known risk factor. For at least 95% of the children who do not manifest a known risk factor one will also need approaches for early hearing loss detection.

13. ERA in the 'difficult-to-test child'

CLINICAL PROBLEM

Until the infant is 4 months of age, the quality of the auditory responses is little dependent on mental development, and only later can auditory behaviour and developmental landmarks differentiate the normal child and the child whose functioning and behaviour are abnormal (Northern & Downs 1984). A battery of audiological tests is applied according to the auditory and mental development of the child. Some children's behaviour and functioning is such that it is difficult to judge their auditory responses to conventional audiometric behavioural tests. Precise audiometric threshold estimation may be desirable in such a child, and objective hearing assessment, using ERA tests, may greatly contribute. Delaying the detection of hearing loss and therapy may deprive the child of critical time in learning auditory skills, and may further compromise the development of his speech and behaviour.

Identification of children who would benefit from ERA is primarily the responsibility of the clinician. It is also important to select appropriate tests in order to obtain the information on the degree of hearing loss in low and high audiometric frequencies. This is important for the correct selection of a hearing aid.

Population

Catlin (1978) reported that 50% of cases of childhood deafness occur within the first year of life, and most of these cases are congenital. Martin (1982) reported the prevalence of hearing loss of 50 dB or more, in all children aged 8 years in the European Economic Community (EEC), as ranging from 0.74–1.48 per 1000.

Behavioural audiometry requires great skill and experience from the tester. In a small proportion of tests, the credibility of the results is questionable, usually because of inadequate co-operation of the child, and reliable pure-tone audiograms are rarely available before a mental age of 4 years.

A wide variety of clinical problems in children of various ages leads to referral for an objective test of hearing, in order to verify the degree of hearing loss and institute the best rehabilitation programme. It has been shown that the time interval between objective hearing estimation with ECochG or ABR and the first 'reliable' pure-tone audiogram may be several years, and that this was obtained at some stage in 31% of 841 tested children (Bellman et al 1984). Some important single features or combinations of salient features in children of various ages, exhibiting both normal intelligence and mental handicap, who may require objective hearing assessment, are listed below:

Mental retardation with or without severe behavioural problems
Behavioural problems only
Cerebral palsy with gross motor involvement
Hyperactivity
Neurological handicap
Speech and language delay or absence
Learning difficulties
Autistic-like state
Severe visual disability
Rubella syndrome
Deafness in various syndromes
Chromosomal abnormalities
Family history of hearing loss
Sudden hearing loss or deterioration

A more extreme group of children can be identified, whose functioning and behaviour are such that they are sometimes untestable, or about whom it is difficult to make a conclusive judgement using standard behavioural audiometric techniques. This group of children is known as the 'difficult-to-test' children, including mentally retarded, brain-damaged or centrally disordered, autistic-like, and deaf-blind children.

Neither mental retardation, nor central auditory disorder, nor autism result, in themselves, in hearing loss, but when behavioural auditory responses suggest hearing loss, or pure-tone audiograms are not credible, these conditions have to be verified. However, it is possible for such children to have peripheral hearing loss. For example, in mental institutions, the prevalence of hearing loss and ear disease ranges from 10 to 45% or higher (Northern & Downs 1984). Brain-damaged, autistic, or hyperactive children who have difficulty in paying attention for any length of time may be difficult to test with conventional audiometric methods; they are prime candidates for ERA.

Some children with neurological handicaps and visual disability have delay of language and of other developmental characteristics. They often fail behavioural audiometric tests and are classified as 'the deaf-blind' child; however, on testing them later, it may appear that some of them have normal hearing (Stein et al 1981). Various eye–ear syndromes, congenital neuromuscular disorders, and rubella can be associated with deafness.

CHOICE OF ERA TESTS

An appropriate behavioural audiometric test is chosen to match the mental development of the child. One has to possess considerable experience and expertise to assess difficult-to-test children. If the auditory responses correspond to the behavioural landmarks, then the hearing is considered normal.

Impedance audiometry in a child of 6 months of age or older is a useful additional test in assessing middle-ear function and acoustic reflexes. The absence of acoustic reflexes suggests hearing loss. However, one should be aware that normal responses may be present in a mild hearing loss with recruitment. Auditory behavioural testing and impedance audiometry may be difficult to attain in 'the difficult-to-test child'. ERA should be used, if necessary, to clarify the hearing level and audiometric contour. However, one should remember that ERA is not a simple procedure, and that precise results depend on the expertise of the tester.

ERA requires minimum gross body movement. Testing with scalp-attached electrodes in natural sleep following feeding is suitable in infants under 4 months of age.

In older children, the investigation is carried out under sedation or general anaesthesia, and testing time becomes an important factor.

Several different types of sedation to induce sleep have been recommended, including, for example, oral and rectal administration of chloral derivatives; a phenobarbital suppository (5 mg/kg body weight) in infants older than 3 months; Vallergan forte syrup (4 mg/kg body weight) administered half an hour before the test; cocktails of chlorpromazine (5 mg) and promethazine (4 mg/5 ml solution administered 1 ml/kg body weight, repeating half of the dose if there is no effect after 20 minutes, and maximally administering another half of the dose if there is still no effect after another 20 minutes). In some difficult-to-test children, the effect of sedation is often inadequate and difficult to predict.

General anaesthesia guarantees very good recording conditions, and the tests are carried out after administering either an intramuscular injection of ketamine or inhalation anaesthesia with halothane (occasionally Ethrane) with nitrous oxide and oxygen. Such anaesthesia enables relatively invasive ECochG using a transtympanic needle electrode.

The clinician has to decide what the most important information is that he wants to obtain, and choose the procedure that avoids a long testing time.

ECochG is a very useful procedure when applied in 'difficult-to-test' children (Fig. 13.1). Assessment of hearing at the level of the cochlea is obtained from the stimulated ear only, and there is no contribution from

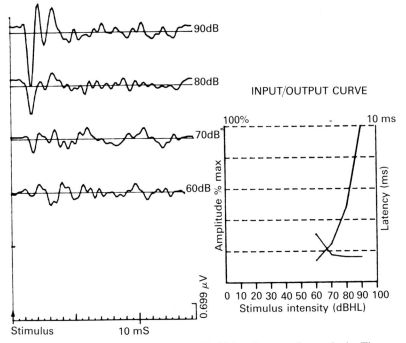

Fig. 13.1 ECochG recording from a 2-year-old child under general anaesthesia. The waveform and amplitude and latency I/O functions show a 'recruiting' type of loss.

the better ear at high-intensity stimulation level when there is a sound cross-over effect. Click-evoked ECochG is the most sensitive test, especially for moderately severe to severe hearing loss, and the correlation with the pure-tone audiogram at 1000, 2000, and 4000 Hz is very good. Correlation between the ECochG threshold and the behavioural threshold in free field in difficult-to-test children was found to be good, although the differences between the two values increased with increase of hearing loss (Bergholtz et al 1977). ECochG is a comparatively quick test, and responses can be obtained in 128 to 256 samples. Its disadvantage is difficulty in assessing hearing at lower frequencies, and the responses correlate best with the hearing level for audiometric frequencies above 1000 Hz.

A comparison of threshold sensitivities in children showed that ECochG threshold is a slightly more sensitive measure of peripheral hearing than ABR (Ryerson & Beagley 1981). However, ABR is a non-invasive test and can be used in a carefully selected, sleeping difficult-to-test child under sedation, without general anaesthesia. General anaesthesia itself does not have a noticeable effect on ABR, but its use should be considered carefully in a child with multiple handicaps. In general, click-evoked ABRs are thought to be slightly less sensitive than ECochG in children with hearing loss; however, ABR is a very important contributory test (Bellman et al

1984). ABR correlates very well with the pure-tone audiometric mean threshold at 1000, 2000, and 4000 Hz, and the contribution to the ABR response from the lower frequencies is greater than in ECochG recording. However, the limitations in assessing hearing at low frequencies remain. Initiation of ABR at the level of the cochlea gives valuable information about peripheral auditory sensitivity. However, ABR may be dependent on a lesion in the brainstem, and abnormal ABR results from children with CNS disorders can be ambiguous (Worthington & Peters 1980).

In order to improve the frequency specificity of ABR for assessment of the clinically important, low audiometric frequency of 500 Hz, some clinicians have advocated short tone pips of 2, 1, 2 ms rise, plateau, and fall duration time. These 500 Hz tone pips can be presented in high-pass or notch-filtered masking noise, assuming that the ABR response is obtained from the unmasked part of the cochlea only. The trough after wave V can be enhanced by expanding the filter at lower frequencies; this causes distortion in the pre-amplifier filter, recording a vertex negative wave SN10 with the latency around 10–14 ms. However, the accuracy of prediction of these responses to low-frequency and low-intensity tone pips has been questioned (Hayes & Jerger 1982).

The middle-latency responses are considered more frequency specific, and by stimulating at a rate 40/s, one can obtain an enhanced response called the 40 Hz response, representing the actual Pa potential of the MLR at about 25 ms. These responses are thought to be recorded even better at low audiometric frequencies, and could be included in assessing them. However, the disadvantage is that the amplitude decreases substantially in a sleeping child, and sedation also decreases the amplitude (Mendel & Goldstein 1971, Shallop & Osterhammel 1983).

The SVR has good hearing-level sensitivity and good frequency specificity, making it an excellent audiometric tool in a co-operating adult. In a difficult-to-test child, however, it is usually unsuitable, because sleep, sedation, and general anaesthesia make the identification of the responses unpredictable.

We may conclude that a combination of tests may be needed to assess the hearing level in both ears and to determine the audiometric contour; relevant tests and their corresponding parameters are shown in Table 13.1.

Table 13.1 ERA tests and parameters for hearing estimation in children

Test	ECochG	ABR	40-Hz MLR
Signal	click ±	click ±	tone pip: 500 Hz
Rate	10–20/s	30/s	40/s
Number of averages	128–256	2048	1024
Filter passband	30–3000 Hz	30–3000 Hz	20–80 Hz

ERA STRATEGIES

A comprehensive assessment of difficult-to-test children requires testing with behavioural audiometry and impedance audiometry, including acoustic reflexes and ERA. The best thresholds from all the tests should be used to estimate the hearing loss.

The task of evaluating the hearing level of both ears and determining which is the better ear and what is the audiometric contour can be facilitated and improved by using ERA.

To some extent, the testing strategy will depend on whether the child can be tested under sedation or requires general anaesthesia. The most difficult-to-test children require general anaesthesia, analogous to that required for minor surgery.

Testing under general anaesthesia in the operating theatre introduces undesirable ambient electrical noise, which should be minimized as much as possible. ECochG, which has the best signal-to-noise ratio, usually gives clearer responses in that environment than ABR, especially in the presence of severe hearing loss. Transtympanic electrocochleography is the quickest response using 128 broad-band click stimuli per recording. The responses are recorded separately from each ear and traced to the threshold. At least two averages should be done at the threshold for surer detection of the response. Drawing the intensity–amplitude function may reveal the type of hearing loss.

ECochG responses obtained at or below 20 dBnHL indicate normal hearing in the 2000–4000 Hz audiometric frequency range. Furthermore, for practical reasons, detailed audiometric contour assessment is not essential. ABR is a useful test in this population, especially in children with CNS disorders. ABR with abnormal morphology and latencies and elevated thresholds can be recorded in the presence of normal peripheral hearing on ECochG (Bellman et al 1984).

Elevated ECochG thresholds to click stimuli suggest a hearing loss, and warrant further audiometric contour assessment with tone pips. Low audiometric frequency at 500 Hz may be assessed using either SN10 or 40-Hz MLR tests. Click-evoked ABR is advisable as a neuro-otological test.

The absence of an ECochG response to 100 dB broad-band click stimulus suggests a severe hearing loss. The correlation between the ECochG threshold and hearing loss gets weaker as the hearing loss increases. In the absence of CAP, the residual hearing of 90–115 dBnHL may be present at high audiometric frequencies in the basal turn, and even more so at the low audiometric frequencies in the apical parts of the cochlea. Assessment of the audiometric contour is desirable in this situation, and testing with tone pips at 2000–1000 Hz may be more revealing in picking up ECochG responses. ABR has similar frequency specificity, but wave V has more weighting from lower frequencies in the cochlea than does the AP of the electrocochleographic response. Therefore, it is prudent to try to estimate the low-frequency hearing loss with tone pip-evoked ABR or SN10. The 40 Hz MLR response at the audiometric frequency of 500 Hz is very desirable. However, in the presence of severe hearing loss, this response has not been sufficiently well evaluated. Furthermore, both MLR and, even more so, SVR are compromised by the general anaesthesia which is necessary to keep difficult-to-test children still. Therefore, SVR is rarely useful as a test in an anaesthetized child.

Hearing assessment with clicks can be done using ABR instead of transtympanic ECochG, especially when sleep is induced by sedation only. In order to economize on the testing time, a binaural stimulation strategy in recording ABR has been recommended (Jerger et al 1984). With this strategy, ABR thresholds reflect the sensitivity of the better ear. It is known that ABR responses evoked by binaural stimulation at equal sensation levels are not smaller than either monaural response (Gerull & Mrowinski 1984). There are some practical advantages with this strategy. If the child wakes up and is not testable following binaural assessment, it may be assumed that the ABR threshold represents the hearing level of the better ear, allowing experimental fitting of the hearing aid on one of the ears at a time.

Overall, it appears that click-evoked ECochG and ABR are the most efficient tests in assessing hearing in the middle range and high audiometric frequencies in difficult-to-test children under general anaesthesia or sedation. Hearing levels at low audiometric frequencies can be estimated by using tone pips with masking techniques and recording ABR and SN10 or 40 Hz MLR.

DIFFERENTIATION OF CONDUCTIVE AND COCHLEAR HEARING LOSS

Impedance audiometry is very helpful in the detection of middle-ear dysfunction. With the conventional low-frequency probe tones of 200–600 Hz, there are limitations in testing young children. However, equipment nowadays can also provide 1000 Hz probe tones, in which the shorter wavelengths compensate for the small ear canals found in neonates, and make testing such patients a practical proposition. In older children with normal middle-ear compliance, the acoustic stapedial reflex may not be elicited as a result of either ossicular fixation in conductive hearing loss, or severe sensorineural hearing loss, making the results of the test noncontributory.

We think that ERA can provide broader audiometric information. ABR techniques and functions may be applied in the same way as for adults. The intensity–amplitude and intensity–latency relationships for CAP, and intensity–latency relationship for ABR wave V, may suggest the type of hearing loss, as shown in Figure 13.2 (see also Chs. 5 and 7).

Bone-conduction techniques for ERA are considered useful and feasible,

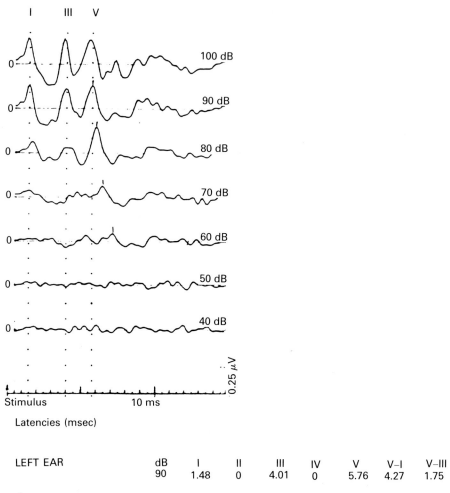

LEFT EAR	dB	I	II	III	IV	V	V–I	V–III
	90	1.48	0	4.01	0	5.76	4.27	1.75

A

Fig. 13.2 ABR recording from 2-year-old child using click stimulation at the rate of 30/s. The I–V inter-peak interval is normal. Both the waveform amplitudes (**A**) and the wave-V latency I/O function (**B**) demonstrate a recruiting pattern. This implies a cochlear lesion.

but the use of stimuli for ECochG and ABR presents some technical difficulties.

ABR IN INVESTIGATION OF NEUROLOGICAL DYSFUNCTION IN CHILDREN

Together with hearing assessment, ABR is applied to the investigation of brainstem dysfunction in difficult-to-test children. Unsuspected abnormal brainstem problems may be revealed through abnormal ABR morphology

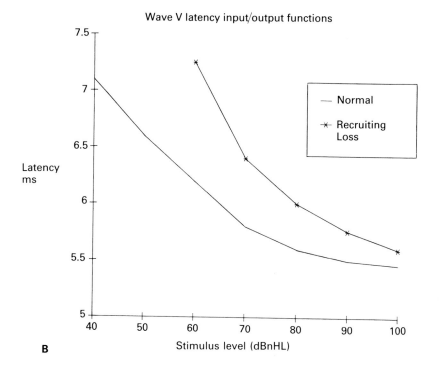

Wave V latency input/output functions

B

and threshold when peripheral hearing is normal according to ECochG. Most anaesthetic agents and drugs do not produce a noticeable effect on ABR in therapeutic doses. However, some anaesthetics, e.g. lignocaine, have been found to prolong the latencies. Numerous conditions may be responsible for abnormal ABR due to brainstem dysfunction in children, and some of these are listed below.

Meningitis and encephalitis
Vasculitis
Raised intracranial pressure
Hypoxia
Tumours
Demyelinating metabolic disorders
Neurodegenerative disorders
Chromosomal disorders

14. ERA in non-organic hearing loss (NOHL)

CLINICAL PROBLEM

A subject may exhibit deliberately false hearing thresholds or have an unconsciously raised threshold of response. Such subjects are categorized as having non-organic hearing loss (NOHL). Adult patients exhibiting NOHL tend to be exaggerators and malingerers, but they commonly exhibit a functional hearing loss which may have been unconsciously elevated; that is, the NOHL may be superimposed on a genuine hearing impairment. Not uncommonly children aged between 6 and 14 years can exhibit NOHL and the cause may generally be traced to family and/or school problems.

Verification of hearing loss and validation of the pure-tone audiogram is of special relevance in dealing with compensation claimants in medicolegal practice. Hearing threshold may be affected by numerous factors, including poor comprehension of the test requirements as a result of low intellectual or linguistic ability, fatigue, and temporary threshold shift due to recent noise exposure.

An important factor in detecting a bogus NOHL is a high initial index of suspicion on the part of the clinician or audiologist. A patient's history, especially in medicolegal cases concerning compensation, may alert the otologist. Suspicion of a claimed NOHL can be based on the patient's behaviour and discrepancies in the results of auditory tests such as pure-tone, speech, and impedance audiometry. Suspicious audiometric findings may include pure-tone and speech reception threshold differences greater than 10 dB and pure-tone thresholds close to or above the acoustic stapedial reflex threshold.

Having suspected the NOHL, one can administer a variety of tests to detect a bogus NOHL. These include the Lombard test, the Von Békésy test, and some other more complicated methods, which, in any case, do not reveal true hearing threshold. Threshold estimation from acoustic reflex measurement is not sufficiently accurate. Stenger's test is useful when there is considerable unilateral NOHL.

The need for more precise assessment of the threshold at audiometric frequencies has drawn attention to ERA, of which SVR is the test of choice. Having suspected a patient of bogus NOHL after observing clinical and audiometric discrepancies, one may use numerous confirmatory tests for detection. Accurate estimation of audiometric threshold is the next stage in assessing NOHL, and ERA has a definite role to play.

ERA TESTS FOR NOHL

ERA tests for threshold estimation depend on subjective judgement of response presence or absence; therefore, proper technical experience is essential. SVR, MLR, ABR, and CAP recorded using electrocochleography can be employed in hearing threshold assessment. However, the tests differ in their frequency specificity, accuracy, and convenience.

SVR is the test of choice for verification of the pure-tone audiogram in order to exclude NOHL in adults and adolescents. This ERA method is the nearest to conventional audiometry. It is frequency specific and relatively insensitive to neurological dysfunction. Monaural stimulation is used. Usually air-conduction testing is done, and bone-conduction testing is rarely required. By testing low frequencies at high intensities, especially with a bone conductor on the skin, one can record a response to a vibro-tactile stimulus. SVR is thought to be enhanced by stimulus-orientated attention, and, therefore, the patient is instructed to pay attention. The deliberate exaggerator usually increases his attention because of anxiety, and SVRs are often very clear in patients who deliberately exaggerate hearing loss.

Using fairly long tone bursts of about 100 ms duration with a rise–fall time of 10 ms, one can construct an audiogram at selected low and high audiometric frequencies.

Stimuli are presented at a rate of 1/2 s, with the number of sweeps ranging from 20 to 40. At least two averages should be recorded at a threshold. Replication at a threshold will help to identify the peaks of the SVR and avoid false-positive response detection. High levels of EEG alpha rhythm make it very difficult to detect SVR reliably in about 5% of cases (Hyde et al 1986).

SVR-ERA is a lengthy procedure, and it is best to limit the number of frequencies tested. However, in most cases an audiogram at 500, 1000, 2000, and 3000 Hz can be estimated within an hour. For assessment, in a medicolegal case of an individual claiming compensation for occupational hearing loss, the frequencies 500, 1000, 2000, and 3000 Hz are essential, as combinations of them have been used to calculate the degree of disability.

Recording MLR using a stimulation rate of 40/s instead of the usual rate of 10/s, one can achieve superimposition of the peaks of MLR and augmentation of the response. When SVR measurement conditions are poor, the 40 Hz MLR gives more reasonable threshold estimates. However, when SVR conditions are good, 40 Hz MLR threshold estimates are the more variable of the two (Hyde et al 1986).

ABRs using clicks and short tone bursts have significant drawbacks as regards frequency specificity, and, therefore, their use in audiometric verification is limited. Some improvement in frequency specificity is possible by using ipsilateral notch masking or high-pass masking derived-response techniques. Only in a few instances where SVR is not obtained is ABR used for detection of NOHL. The averaging time is comparable to that of SVR.

Transtympanic ECochG gives the best signal-to-noise ratio. However, its limitation as regards frequency specificity is similar to that of ABR. Being an invasive procedure, ECochG should be avoided in assessment of NOHL in adults, especially in compensation claimants.

ERA TESTING STRATEGIES

ERA, being an objective test, is naturally useful in this situation because it can give an estimate of hearing loss. Because of its good frequency specificity, SVR is the test of choice. But other tests can be used in school-age children and adults when conditions for SVR recording are poor, or SVR results require corroboration. ABR and MLR tests can be used alternatively.

If the ERA results are better than conventional audiometric thresholds, then functional hearing loss is shown. When the audiometric threshold is greater than the SVR threshold by 15 dB or more on any of the frequencies, then NOHL is strongly suggested (Hyde et al 1986). Following ERA testing, the patient is re-instructed, and an attempt is made to obtain another pure-tone audiogram for revalidation. With this strategy of SVR, the other less accurate tests for detection and threshold evaluation of NOHL may perhaps be omitted and the testing time saved.

Sometimes NOHL must be ruled out in young children who give a hearing loss on pure-tone audiogram greater than expected from clinical observation. The problem may be resolved by tracing the threshold with broad-band click-evoked ABR. If the ABR thresholds are within normal limits, one should attempt to persuade the child to give true pure-tone thresholds.

If the ERA tests are consistent with and support the results of the conventional audiometric tests, the suspicion of functional hearing loss should be reviewed. The SVR thresholds are within 10 dB of the pure-tone audiogram thresholds.

When ERA thresholds are higher than conventional audiometric thresholds, the ERA tests are non-contributory. In a small proportion of cases, the ERA thresholds may be elevated for unknown reasons, e.g. poor recording conditions, high EEG rhythmic activity, or high myogenic activity, especially in an anxious patient. In the latter situation, a dose of diazepam may improve the recording.

An SVR-ERA threshold considerably worse than that obtained by pure-tone audiogram may occur in a situation of deliberate concealment of true hearing loss.

When necessary, several ERA tests can be used to corroborate the results of estimated hearing level.

ERA testing strategies for medicolegal assessment

Frequency-specific responses are best obtained using SVR, which is the test of choice for NOHL. It is desirable to use SVR in audiometric assessment of compensation claims in medicolegal cases in order to confirm that the pure-tone audiogram satisfactorily represents the hearing loss. Discrepancies between routine audiometric tests such as pure-tone and speech result, pure-tone and speech reception thresholds, differing by more than 10 dB, pure-tone audiogram thresholds close to or above the acoustic reflex threshold, all require verification with SVR.

SVR testing provides, to some degree, an objective estimate of the hearing level and can be used as a target. When the audiometric threshold and SVR threshold agree within 10 dB, the behavioural threshold is confirmed. When the audiometric threshold is greater than the SVR threshold by 15 dB or more on any of the frequencies, then NOHL should be strongly suspected (Hyde et al 1986). Every effort should be made to resolve the discrepancies between thresholds obtained by SVR and pure-tone audiogram.

In conclusion, the accuracy of SVR depends on technical experience and judgement, as the assessment of the threshold is subjective. In a small proportion of patients, where SVR recording is problematic, other non-invasive ERA tests can be used. The better frequency specificity of 40 Hz MLR makes it preferable to ABR, although the latter is adequate for the purpose of detection of NOHL.

15. ERA in neuro-otologic diagnosis

CLINICAL PROBLEM

The ERA tests are valuable in differentiating cochlear from retrocochlear hearing loss, confirming lesions, and detecting unsuspected retrocochlear pathology (Robinson & Rudge 1983). The more common problems referred to neuro-otologists which may require ERA testing are listed below:

Unilateral hearing loss
Hearing loss with uncertain diagnosis
Unilateral tinnitus
Vertigo suspected from VIIIth nerve or brainstem lesion
Cranial nerve disorders, e.g. nerves V and VII
Ataxia and neurological disorders
Monitoring effect of treatment
Per-operative monitoring of auditory function
Evaluation of electrical cochlear stimulation

CHOICE OF ERA TESTS

The testing strategies depend on the clinical symptomatology and suspected site of lesion. Of all ERA tests, ABR is the most suitable test for this purpose. MLR and ECochG may contribute to establishing the site of the lesion in a specific situation; however, each test on its own is less valuable than in combination. Table 15.1 shows the effect of various pathologies on the EPs.

Standardization of ERA test procedures for neuro-otological strategies is desirable. This is especially relevant for ABR, which is the most important diagnostic tool, and the clinician has to rely on specific diagnostic parameters. ERA tests and recommended parameters for neuro-otological testing are shown in Table 15.2.

ECochG is used in neuro-otological testing in order to establish the latency of the potential generated at the cochlear nerve site. It becomes especially helpful when wave I of ABR cannot be recorded in cases of moderate and severe hearing losses. The waveform of the compound action potential and SP reflect the pathophysiologic status in the cochlear, and clearest responses

Table 15.1 EP parameters alterable by various pathologies

EP	Hair cell loss	Hydrops (Ménière's disease)	VIIIth nerve lesion	CP-angle lesion	Brainstem lesion	Cortical lesion
SVR	threshold	threshold	threshold	threshold	threshold***	threshold waveform
MLR	threshold	threshold	threshold	threshold	threshold*** waveform latency	normal
ABR	threshold waveform latency	threshold latency TWV**	threshold waveform latency amplitude IPIs	threshold waveform latency amplitude IPIs	threshold*** waveform latency amplitude IPIs	normal
ECochG CAP	threshold waveform latency	threshold	threshold* waveform latency	threshold*	normal	normal
SP	amplitude	amplitude	amplitude	normal	normal	normal
CM	amplitude	variable	normal	normal	normal	normal

* with involvement of the end-organ and/or intracapalicular tumours
** TWV = Travelling wave velocity ABR measures (see p. 110)
*** Unilateral lesions do not cause threshold changes unless the generator of the response, used to estimate threshold is affected by the lesion. Bilateral or large-midline lesions can cause threshold changes in all responses rostral to the lesion.

Table 15.2 ERA tests and parameters

Test	ECochG	ABR	MLR
Stimulus	click alternating	click alternating	click rarefaction
Intensity	80–110 dB	70–100 dB	70–80 dB
Rate	10/s	10/s	<10/s
Number of averages	128–256	2048	512–1024
Filter pass-band	10–3000 Hz	100–3000 Hz	30–300 Hz

are obtained at high intensity click stimuli. However, some investigators found this test on its own of little use in acoustic tumour detection, or in differentiating between cochlear and retrocochlear pathologies. Testing conditions, stimulus intensities, repetition rate, and polarity are the same as for ABR, but the recording band-pass filters are not the same. For ECochG, a broader band-pass filter of 10–3000 Hz is used.

When ABR is used for neuro-otological testing, the aim is to obtain clearly defined peaks of the waves, so that the latencies can be measured accurately. For CNS lesions, useful diagnostic information may be obtained from a comparison of both ipsilateral and contralateral (to the side of stimulation) ABRs. Hence, bilateral recordings should be used routinely. Monaural stimulation is used and the results compared with the normative data. However, if the other ear is not affected, it may act as a partial control for age and sex.

High intensity clicks are used in order to obtain all components of the ABR. Clicks of 80 dBnHL may be used in the presence of hearing loss up to 40 dBnHL at 4000 Hz. For greater hearing loss, a click stimulus of 90–100 dBnHL is more appropriate.

Stimuli at a rate of approximately 10/s do not affect the latencies and waveform of ABR; therefore, a rate of 10/s is used in a standard neuro-otological test procedure. At higher repetition rates, especially in the presence of high frequency hearing loss, the components of the ABR degrade, wave I in particular, and, hence, compromise the measurement of inter-peak intervals. The auditory system may be stressed by stimulating at higher rates of 50–70/s, and this may elicit more subtle abnormalities. Abnormal responses may suggest a retrocochlear disorder (Shanon et al 1981, Pratt et al 1981). Employing alternating polarity clicks seems to be a rational way of testing, because electrical polarity does not always correspond to acoustic polarity at the eardrum (Salt 1982). In the presence of steep high frequency hearing loss, the latency differences between stimulation with condensation and rarefaction clicks may be considerable (see p. 93).

An abnormal MLR may reveal brainstem lesions. It can be recorded in addition to the ABR, using the same electrode derivation. Usually rarefaction click stimuli of high intensity, at a rate of less than 10/s, are used, and the recording band-pass is 30–300 Hz.

INTERPRETATION OF ERA TESTS

A proportion of false-positive and false-negative data is possible, and, therefore, ERA should be interpreted in conjunction with other investigations. Accurate pure-tone audiograms and impedance audiometry are desirable prior to ERA tests. For the neuro-otologic population, criteria pointing to abnormalities in ERA tests are based on assessing the morphology of the responses, the prolongation of the latencies, and abnormal amplitude ratios.

Differentiation of cochlear from retrocochlear lesions relies mainly on ABR. A large proportion of neuro-otologic patients have mild or normal hearing on the pure-tone audiogram. The useful diagnostic parameters for detecting and interpreting abnormal ABRs are listed in Table 15.3.

An interaural latency difference of greater than 0.3 ms is considered abnormal, providing there is no evidence of hearing loss due to middle ear

Table 15.3 ERA diagnostic parameters

ABR	MLR	ECochG
Abnormal waveform	Abnormal waves	Abnormal AP
Latency of wave V (LV)		L–I function
Interaural latency difference (IT 5)		A–I function
Inter-peak interval (IPI I–V)		SP/AP ratio
Interaural difference of I–V intervals		
Amplitude ratio V/I		

pathology. The inter-peak intervals are independent of conductive hearing loss, and separation into I–III and III–V intervals can sometimes suggest a lesion in the lower or upper brainstem.

The subjective assessment of ABR morphology is valuable; selective absence of late waves and 50% reversal of V/I amplitude ratio are good indications of a retrocochlear lesion. The V/I amplitude ratio is a less valuable parameter for retrocochlear assessment in the presence of cochlear hearing loss.

The MLR can provide additional information, as it has been reported that there is abnormal wave morphology in some patients with multiple sclerosis (Robinson & Rudge 1980).

Abnormally enhanced SPs, recorded by ECochG, support a clinical diagnosis of Ménière's disease. Also, AP latencies recorded at the cochlear level in cases of moderate to severe hearing loss, together with the inter-peak intervals and wave V latency of ABR, can help to separate cochlear from retrocochlear lesions.

The latencies and amplitudes can be measured, and normative values should be established for every clinic. A typical diagnostic evaluation of a mean and two standard deviations predicts a false-positive rate of 5%. However, a greater percentage of false-positive errors can be accepted when using ABR as a screening test for patient selection and for further, more expensive or invasive, diagnostic radiological CT and MRI testing. Also, ABR can reduce the number of other audiometric tests and improve site-of-lesion diagnosis.

INVESTIGATION OF UNILATERAL HEARING LOSS

Clinical problem

A patient with unilateral or asymmetric sensorineural hearing loss should be suspected of acoustic tumour unless the history is clearly associated with trauma or acute infection. The suspect group includes patients with sudden onset of symptoms and those whose initial presentation is suggestive of Ménière's disease. Shaia & Sheehy (1976) reported a 0.8% tumour occurrence in 1220 cases of sudden unilateral hearing loss, but only 15–17% of tumours present with this symptom (Meyerhoff 1981, Morrison 1975). This situation requires screening tests by which patients can be selected for elaborate or invasive procedures. In acoustic tumour, auditory symptoms are the first to develop in most cases, and, therefore, hearing evaluation should initiate the screening programme.

Tests

Generally, speech-reception threshold and speech-discrimination scores have poor performance as differential diagnostic measures, and correlate only weakly with tumour size in confirmed cases (Johnson 1979, Eggermont et al 1980). Many other supra-threshold auditory tests, including ABLB, SISI, and tone decay, have been claimed to have diagnostic value, but critical appraisal of the performance of these tests has revealed contradictory patterns of results and unacceptable error rates (Saunders et al 1974, Clemis & Mastricola 1976, Johnson 1979). Devotees of battery approaches frequently ignore the implications for net error rates when many tests are combined.

Acoustic reflex testing is objective and merits consideration as a component of the screening battery, provided the hearing loss is mild. The reflex is absent or decays in about 80% of patients with tumours (Saunders et al 1974). Even for small tumours, all 6 in Johnson's series (1979) and 4 out of 7 in Selters & Brackmann's series (1977) were abnormal on this test. However, many patients with cochlear disorders show absent reflexes, as do those with minor middle-ear disease, so the predictive value of absent reflexes is questionable (Cashman & Rossman 1983).

As regards vestibular testing, 40% of small tumours have caloric responses within the normal range, but of all tumours a reduced response is found in 82% of cases (Lintchicum et al 1979). However, 23% of cases with non-tumour diagnoses have reduced caloric responses (Selters & Brackmann 1979), so this test has limited specificity.

ABR testing has been reported to be an excellent test for acoustic tumour detection, being positive in 90–100% of confirmed cases. A selective loss of late waves is a positive indication of a retrocochlear lesion. An important caveat is that a significant proportion of cases requiring screening tests such as ABR may have a severe hearing loss, and in many such cases the ABR will be absent when the suspected ear is stimulated. In this instance, the test will not contribute to the differential diagnosis of cochlear or peripheral nerve lesion.

The ABR parameters used most often in the detection of acoustic tumours are the absolute latency of wave V, the interaural difference among waves V (IT 5), and the inter-peak latency among waves I–V (IPI I–V). Prolongation of these parameters are the criteria for acoustic-tumour detection. Wave V latency increases strongly and non-linearly with 4000 Hz pure-tone loss, and a correction factor has to be applied in order to reduce a false-positive error rate (see Ch. 8). The interaural latency difference IT 5 is more specific than latency of wave V parameter, because the non-tumorous ear acts as a partial control for sex and age. IPI I–V is less sensitive to hearing loss and may contribute to a more accurate overall interpretation.

However, in a considerable number of patients with severe high frequency loss, wave I is not identifiable in up to 50% of cases, and we have to rely on IT 5, or, alternatively, wave I can be measured by trans-tympanic or endomeatal ECochG (Fig. 15.1). Even with its current limitations, the ABR test is generally considered to be a very valuable procedure for acoustic tumour detection. Its use can improve and abbreviate the audiometric test battery. Audiometric investigation can be limited to pure-tone audiometry, impedance audiometry with the acoustic stapedial reflex test, and ABR. When ABR results are inconclusive, especially when there

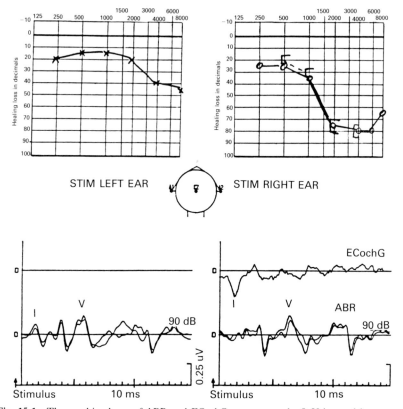

Fig. 15.1 The combined use of ABR and ECochG to measure the I–V interval in a case of asymmetric hearing loss. The right-side I–V interval is abnormal. The patient had a right-side meningioma.

is severe hearing loss, vestibular testing may become relevant. However, there has yet to be a detailed analysis of caloric test results in a large group of non-contributory ABR and in proven cases of false-negative ABR. Accurate pure-tone audiometry is desirable prior to ABR testing and interpretation, especially if good control of false-positive errors by latency correction is required, as opposed to routine use of electrocochleography to clarify wave I and IPI I–V.

As the sole test for detection of acoustic tumours, ECochG appears to be of limited value. ECochG supplies additional information by clarifying the latency of wave I, and is helpful when other parameters indicate a tumour. Therefore, for cases with strong clinical indication of a tumour, but with questionable ABR, ECochG can be helpful. Features of ECochG associated with a tumour include abnormal width of AP, abnormal amplitude of SP, and considerable difference between subjective and ECochG thresholds. ABR results, provided they are definite, override other audiometric tests as determinants of subsequent investigation.

ERA testing strategies

Assuming that all patients under investigation for a retrocochlear lesion are candidates for ABR, four situations can face the otologist: (i) the ABR is positive, (ii) borderline positive or questionable, (iii) negative, and (iv) non-contributory. Radiological assessment of structural abnormalities of the IAM and CP angle must take account of these functional findings.

Our suggested schemes are merely guidelines illustrating our view of the way ABR and radiological studies may be combined effectively.

Definite positive ABR is followed by contrast-enhanced CT, which, if negative, is followed by Air CT or magnetic resonance imaging (MRI).

Questionable and non-contributory ABR lead to the same test sequence in most cases when a tumour is suspected.

If ABR results are definitely negative, as expected in most cases of asymmetric sensorineural hearing loss, then CT studies are not usually indicated. The case should be reassessed on clinical grounds, to determine whether further investigations or subsequent review, including a repeat ABR, is warranted. Non-invasive but more expensive, MRI may replace CT studies in the future in some cases.

ERA IN INVESTIGATION OF PATIENTS WITH OTOLOGIC SYMPTOMS AND CRANIAL NERVE DYSFUNCTION

Auditory and vestibular symptoms, especially unilateral, as well as dysfunction of other cranial nerves, in particular, the Vth and VIIth, may reveal a lesion in the CP angle or in the brainstem.

Sensorineural hearing loss

False-positive results for acoustic tumours have been reported by many authors when investigating a unilateral sensorineural hearing loss. It should be noted that the false-positive rate obtained in any study will depend greatly upon the pattern and severity of hearing losses included in the study sample. Josey et al (1984) investigated 902 patients with various aetiologies of sensorineural hearing loss due to ototoxic drugs, presbyacusis, hereditary loss, etc. They used IT 5 as their main criterion of normality. ABR was normal in 87.3%, but in 12.7% of cases, ABR was interpreted as abnormal, although there were no other findings to confirm additional retrocochlear pathology. It should be noted that ABR abnormalities with no audiologically detectable retrocochlear pathology can exist.

It should also be noted that even when the audiometric threshold is so great that one would not expect to record an ABR, the test may, nevertheless, provide useful information.

Consider a case of severe unilateral loss on the left side. Stimulation of the ear (with appropriate masking in the non-tested ear) gives no ABR on either the left or right side. Stimulation of the right ear gives a normal ABR response for all components recorded from the right side, and, on the left side, all the central components of the ABR are within normal limits for a contralateral response. The implication here is that if the left side central components, when receiving input from the right side, are normal, then the lesion is most probably restricted to the peripheral region on the right side.

Another example is a case of bilateral hearing loss of, say, 60 dB HTL. If the ABR recorded from both sides, (a) has normal amplitudes, latencies and waveform, or (b) the first three waves have normal amplitudes, latencies, and waveform, this, respectively, would imply bilateral CNS lesions at (i) a level rostral to the brainstem, or (ii) a level corresponding to the generators of wave V. In case (i), further testing with MLRs and SVRs would be indicated to locate the level of the disorder.

CNS lesions, unless they are large and in the midline, or bilateral, do not, in general, cause pure-tone audiometric losses.

Tinnitus

In patients with unilateral tinnitus, an acoustic tumour should not be ruled out. Sheehy (1979) considered that tinnitus is often the earliest tumour symptom, and it is worth doing an ABR test in such cases. In subjects who have cochlear hearing loss and those who have normal hearing with tinnitus of unknown aetiology, ABR appears normal. Tinnitus does not seem to be associated with any particular electrocochleographic feature (Graham 1981).

Monitoring effects of drugs

During recent years several reports have been published on the effect of some drugs, including lignocaine, tocainide, and phenytoin, on tinnitus, and their intravenous administration effect on the ABR. It has been suggested that intravenous administration of lignocaine may be used to divide patients into responders and non-responders, with a view to further treatment with orally administered drugs. It is hoped that recording of the auditory-evoked potentials will allow a more rational management of tinnitus patients. Lenarz (1985) found that in a group of 24 patients in whom reduction of tinnitus was noticed, 10 had a reversible prolongation of I–V on the ABR, indicating a retrocochlear site of drug action. Experimental studies show that ABR changes correlate positively with the dose of the drug (Lenarz et al 1987).

Facial nerve disorders

Acute peripheral facial palsy

Abnormal ABRs have been reported in some patients with Ramsay Hunt syndrome who exhibited facial palsy, vesicular erruption, and auditory and vestibular symptoms suggesting retrocochlear involvement (Abramovich & Prasher 1986). Acute inflammation of the neural and perineural structures of the VIIth nerve, the adjacent VIIIth nerve, and possibly the surface of the brainstem, caused by the neurotropic virus *Varicella zoster*, could be a factor in the underlying process of desynchronization and poor conduction. Such conditions may cause prolonged interwave intervals of the ABR components and abnormalities of wave morphology. The striking feature of the abnormalities in these patients was the prolongation of the latencies of waves III and V, with preservation of wave I, which clearly suggests retrocochlear involvement. In all patients tested, abnormalities were on the affected side. When retested 6 months later, after clinical recovery, ABRs appeared within normal limits.

Viral, vascular, and polyneuropathic causes have been suggested as aetiological factors in acute idiopathic peripheral facial palsy, otherwise known as Bell's palsy. Several reports have indicated abnormal ABRs in patients with Bell's palsy, and the incidence varied from 6.7 to as high as 25% (Maurizi et al 1987, Rosenhall et al 1983, Uri et al 1984, Shanon et al 1985).

Wave V is most commonly affected, and IPI I–V and IPI III–V are prolonged. Pratt et al (1981) used a high stimulation rate in order to stress the auditory pathway, and they found abnormally prolonged IPIs. Ben-David et al (1986) compared diabetic and non-diabetic patients with Bell's palsy, finding that in the diabetic group the incidence of abnormally prolonged IPI I–V and IPI III–V was significantly greater. Uri et al (1984) investigated Bell's palsy in diabetics, finding abnormally prolonged IPIs only in patients with peripheral neuropathies. Although Maurizi et al (1987), using a 2-SD criterion, reported prolonged latencies of wave V in 10% of patients with Bell's palsy (6.7% using a 3-SD criterion), they thought that ABR abnormalities were not pathogonomonic of Bell's palsy.

Hemifacial spasm

Abnormal ABRs have been reported in hemifacial spasm and its associated compression effect by the loops of the vessels (see p. 121).

Progressive facial nerve palsy

Tumours of the facial nerve originating in the CP-angle may produce ABR changes similar to those produced by acoustic tumours.

Unilateral facial pain and trigeminal neuralgia

Various big tumours in the cerebello-pontine angle can cause facial pain, but these tumours are associated with normal audiometric thresholds. Nevertheless, an abnormal ABR may be recorded as a result of pressure effect on the auditory nerve or the brainstem. When such a tumour is suspected, one should think of ABR testing.

Abnormal ABRs for both ipsilateral and contralateral sides have been observed in trigeminal neuralgia. Moller and Moller (1986) explained bilateral changes of ABR as the result of the vascular loops of the anterior inferior cerebellar artery, and sometimes of the superior cerebellar arteries, pressing on the VIIth nerve and lower brainstem in the region of the cochlear nucleus or trapezoid body. Because the auditory fibres cross at this level to the opposite side, ABR changes on the contralateral side can be expected.

Trigeminal neuralgia could be a manifestation of MS, and when this disorder is suspected, ABR and MLR may be of value.

Dizzy patients

Dizziness can be a manifestation of peripheral or central vestibular lesion as in multiple sclerosis, degenerative vascular lesions, and tumours, all of which may be associated with auditory dysfunction. Abnormal ABRs suggest the involvement of the retrocochlear auditory pathway. In a group of 974 patients diagnosed as suffering from vertigo of unknown aetiology, only 1.1% exhibited abnormal ABRs in the absence of any clinically detectable retrocochlear lesion (Josey et al 1984).

Ménière's disease

In most cases, the diagnosis of Ménière's disease is made solely on the basis of history and audiometry. In some unclear cases, in order to support the diagnosis, special investigations may be revealing; here ABR and ECochG are useful tests. Ménière's disease is characterized by cochlear dysfunction, and ABRs are expected to be negative for retrocochlear lesions. Josey et al (1984) investigated 1308 patients with diagnoses of unilateral or bilateral

Ménière's disease. Of these, 96.2% exhibited true-negative ABRs, while 3.8% exhibited abnormal ABRs consistent with a retrocochlear lesion. A positive ABR test requires further investigations, including a CT scan, in order to exclude a true-positive retrocochlear lesion.

ECochG is a valuable test in the patient suspected of having Ménière's disease. An abnormally enhanced SP has been found in endolymphatic

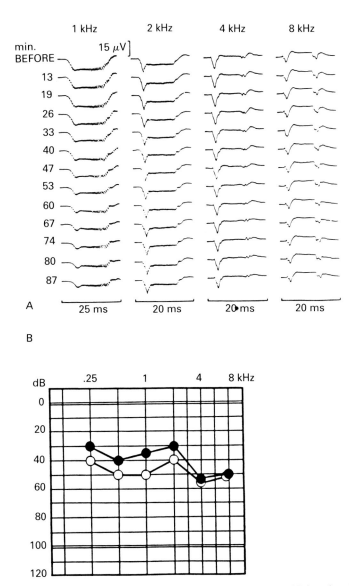

Fig. 15.2 ECochG recorded during a glycerol-dehydration test. The SP is reduced in amplitude as the patient is dehydrated. (After Dauman et al 1988).

hydrops, and the SP correlates well with Ménière's disease. Therefore, the SP can be used to support the provisional diagnosis, especially in a less typical clinical presentation. It has been reported that patients who were totally asymptomatic on the day of testing had normal SP on the endomeatal electrocochleogram (Ferraro et al 1985). Ferraro and his associates suggested that ECochG should be done when the patient is experiencing symptoms, especially hearing loss and aural fullness or pressure.

According to Gibson et al (1983), with mild hearing loss of less than 40 dB HTL, no obvious abnormality was apparent in the click-evoked SP/AP ratio with transtympanic ECochG. However, for losses greater than 40 db HTL, a clear separation emerged between the Ménière's disease group and the sensory group. The SP/AP ratio of 30% provided a diagnostic dividing mark between sensory damage of the cochlea and Ménière's disease. However, there was still a large overlap between the data from Ménière's disease patients and data from normal subjects. The SP complex is much better recorded in Ménière's disease with tone bursts of 10–20 ms duration at 1000 or 2000 Hz, and this stimulus can reveal abnormally enhanced SP when responses to click stimuli are not revealing. The SP/AP ratio with 1000 or 2000 Hz tone bursts is less appropriate than stimulation with clicks, because the AP generation is poor from the apical cochlear region. Some patients with Ménière's disease do not show a pathologic SP or SP/AP ratio, which could be due to progressive deterioration of the hair cells, or to a limited degree of hydrops.

The glycerol-dehydration test has been used long in diagnosing the presence of endolymphatic hydrops. Dauman et al (1988) investigated 50 patients with Ménière's disease, reporting that SP, in response to tone bursts at low frequencies of 1000 and 2000 Hz, decreased in 59% of Ménière's disease patients, whereas subjective hearing improved in only 29% of a subset of those cases (Fig. 15.2). It seems that the use of ECochG together with the monitoring of SP improves the sensitivity of the glycerol-dehydration test for the detection of endolymphatic hydrops.

Thornton & Farrell (1989) reported an objective detection of endolymphatic hydrops with non-invasive ABR technique. They used a derived-response technique initially, and later a simpler, clinical, high-pass masking technique, to estimate the travelling wave velocity (TWV) at different points along the cochlear partition. The travelling wave velocity appears to increase in cases of endolymphatic hydrops (see p. 110).

16. ERA in investigation of neurological disorders

MULTIPLE SCLEROSIS

Clinical problem

The clinical diagnosis of multiple sclerosis is made on the evidence of two or more lesions in the CNS and the exclusion of all other possible causes. Clinically, MS is characterized by exacerbation and remission of symptoms, and the disease's diagnosis is classified into definite, probable, and possible.

ABR and MLR confirm lesions in the CNS in a high proportion of cases. These tests can also detect unsuspected lesions, which is their main value for the clinician in making the diagnosis. It should be noted that visual-evoked potentials (VEP) and somatosensory-evoked potentials (SEP) reveal silent lesions more frequently than does ABR. For many patients who present with symptoms indicating a single lesion, evoked-potential measurements can demonstrate subclinical abnormalities in areas other than the presenting symptom, and thereby clarify the diagnosis.

ERA tests and strategies

Patients with clinical evidence of brainstem lesion at the time of recording have a higher proportion of ABR and MLR abnormalities than do those who do not show brainstem disorders (see Chs. 7 and 9). Among the latter group, however, some investigators describe abnormal ABR in 20–50% of patients (Chiappa & Ropper 1982).

The particular diagnostic value of using evoked potentials, including ABR, is in detecting silent lesions in patients for whom the diagnosis is uncertain.

Rudge (1983) has suggested that it is worth recording MLR, in addition to ABR. In a group of patients with definite multiple sclerosis, many patients with abnormal ABR also have abnormal MLR, and in about 12% of patients with normal ABR, the MLR was abnormal. In the less than definite group of MS patients, the results are similar to those with a definite diagnosis of MS.

A useful clinical procedure is to test, and then raise the patient's body temperature by 1°C, and retest. The increase in temperature causes further abnormalities in previously abnormal responses and can reveal previously silent lesions.

Bilateral recording of ABR should be done, as it can reveal lesions of the crossing pathways from an analysis of the contralateral response.

BRAIN TUMOURS

Abnormalities of ABR, MLR, and SVR are well documented in CNS tumours. However, normal auditory evoked potentials may be found in cases which clinically manifest a tumour. This is not surprising, as it is known that even fairly large CNS tumours can leave the auditory pathway intact.

Several reports have suggested using ABR to monitor the response to treatment of the tumours (Nodar et al 1984), and to detect the effect of potentially neurotoxic therapy on auditory function (Kingston et al 1986).

DIFFUSE LESIONS

Our clinical experience has revealed cases of retrocochlear pathologies which are reflected in abnormal ABRs, but which are audiologically and clinically silent. Cases of infiltrating, rather than space-occupying, lesions; diffuse degenerative vascular conditions; and sometimes barotrauma cases involving decompression accidents whilst diving can all exhibit ABR abnormalities whilst also exhibiting normal audiometric findings. Of course, depending on the exact sites of the lesions involved, various degrees of hearing loss can also occur in such cases.

COMA

Clinical problem

There is a need for objective assessment and monitoring of the brainstem function in a comatose patient. The ABR has been suggested as a test for that purpose, and its value has been explored in cases of metabolic coma, poisoning with CNS depressants, severe head injury, and brain death. ABR has also been applied in the prognosis of coma, especially after head injury, and in the determination of death.

Technical expertise is very important and the interpretation of the results should be in the context of other clinical data. Otoscopic examination is essential prior to ABR, especially in cases of head injury. Abnormalities in the external and middle ear, and fractures of the petrous bone that cause severe hearing loss may affect the interpretation of the ABR.

ERA tests, strategies, and results

Many pharmacological agents, including CNS depressants, e.g. tricyclic antidepressants and barbiturates, can produce abnormal brainstem function on clinical examination, but ABR may not be affected.

Normal ABR can be recorded in patients in metabolic coma (Starr & Achor 1975), as distinguished from those with severe structural brainstem disorder. However, normal ABRs have been reported in paralysed patients with brainstem infarction, suggesting that the auditory pathway has not been damaged (Chiappa 1983).

Hall et al (1985) studied 200 comatose brain-injured patients in intensive care units (ICU), finding that in 85% of cases the recording was adequate. Bone-conduction ABR was valuable when there was middle-ear involvement. Practically, however, the degree of hearing loss following head injury cannot be established, and the hearing may be completely destroyed, imposing limitations on the ABR interpretation. The ABR is valuable as a predictor of the outcome of the case and correlates well with subjective clinical evaluation and the assignment of a Glasgow Coma Score (Brewer & Resnick 1984).

A normal ABR excludes brain death. However, the absence of the ABR is inconclusive, because such factors as severe hearing loss and electrical artefacts in the ICU may compromise the interpretation of the recording. It is an informative test, but does not have absolute diagnostic value, and, therefore, it has not been included as a criterion for establishing brain death.

17. Monitoring auditory evoked potentials during neuro-otologic surgery

CLINICAL PROBLEM

Intra-operative monitoring of CM and AP can record objectively the results of stapedectomy operations at every step of the procedure.

Intra-operative monitoring of cochlear potentials, in particular the SP, has been suggested, in cases of endolymphatic sac decompression and in drainage operations for Ménière's disease, in order to record the effective reduction of SP.

In an effort to preserve hearing, intra-operative monitoring of cochlear and brainstem potentials has been used in neuro-otologic surgery.

Continuous monitoring provides feedback about the condition of the auditory nerve and the auditory pathway in the brainstem, and may identify the mechanism causing loss of response during suboccipital operations for CP-angle tumours, during retrolabyrinthine or retrosigmoid vestibular nerve section, and when the neurosurgeon moves the vessels during microvascular decompression procedures of the facial, trigeminal, and vestibular nerves.

Vascular compromise, especially to the cochlea, can be detected during surgical procedures. Monitoring changes in the latencies of the ABR allows surgeons to modify their techniques, for example, in retraction and surgical manipulation of the brain. The sooner they are notified of the changes, the more effectively they can control the responses. This is particularly relevant when procedures are aimed at preservation of hearing. However, in spite of the immediate preservation of the ECochG potentials, in a proportion of cases the hearing may deteriorate postoperatively as a result of various mechanisms, especially vascular compromise.

Small tumours are harder to diagnose than large ones, but easier to remove; the operation causes fewer deaths, less morbidity, and less residual neurological deficit; the facial nerve often can be spared; and in up to 30% of cases, the hearing can be preserved. In a small study by the National Hospitals for Nervous Diseases, 5 out of the 7 patients with tumours of less than 1.5 cm had their hearing preserved, but 15 out of 17 patients with tumours greater than 1.5m became deaf (Prasher et al 1987, Sabin et al 1987).

CHOICE OF ERA TESTS

The effects of general anaesthesia and continuous stimulation should be taken into consideration when choosing the EP for intra-operative monitoring, and early EPs are more suitable for that reason.

General anaesthesia depresses the activity of the CNS, and the kind of general anaesthesia is of particular importance when choosing an EP for intra-operative monitoring. Lader & Norris (1969) showed that the EP components appearing after 50 ms are significantly affected by nitrous oxide. However, early auditory-evoked potentials, including ECochG and ABR, are not affected significantly, in man, by commonly used anaesthetics, such as thiopentone, nitrous oxide, and halothane (Duncan et al 1979). Neuromuscular blocking agents, such as succinylcholine and pancuronium bromide, used prior to intubation also do not affect the ABR or MLR (Harker et al 1977, Kileny 1983). A considerable drop in body temperature during anaesthesia may prolong the latencies of the ABR and MLR, and have a confounding effect on the responses.

Another essential requirement of intra-operative monitoring is repetitive stimulation, and habituation may affect the response. Picton et al (1976) have demonstrated that the late vertex cortical potentials decline with repeated stimulation, but the MLR and ABR do not.

The early EPs are used in neuro-otologic surgery to measure both hearing sensitivity and the condition of the brainstem when necessary. Arterial hypotension, hypocarbia, and, especially, surgical manoeuvres may affect the ABR (Grundy et al 1981).

ECochG is a very sensitive indicator of the cochlear function, and, in particular, may detect hydrops in Ménière's disease when the SP/AP ratio is measured. Reduction of the endolymphatic pressure during the operation of endolymphatic sac drainage may be reflected in ECochG as a reduction of SP amplitude.

Both ECochG and ABR are useful in acoustic tumour surgery to preserve hearing. However, transtympanic ECochG gives a better resolution and uses less stimulation, hence giving more rapid feedback on changes in cochlear function than does ABR. Recording of the cochlear function is compromised further by the presence of a hearing loss in acoustic tumours and by ambient noise in the operating theatre.

ABR is of some value when more rostral changes are monitored during neuro-otologic surgery, especially latencies of brainstem components such as intervals I–III, I–V.

ERA MONITORING METHODS

Ensuring the stability of the electrodes during the surgical operation is essential. ECochG is recorded using an insulated transtympanic needle electrode, which is placed through the inferior part of the tympanic membrane to rest on the promontory and secured. However, a ball-type electrode put into the niche of the round window through a myringotomy incision or small tympanotomy is much more stable (Sabin et al 1987). The wire from the electrode is secured with wax to the canal wall. A second reference needle electrode is securely inserted into the ipsilateral ear lobe.

The ABR is recorded between a needle electrode inserted in the scalp at the vertex and the ipsilateral ear lobe. A compromise can be achieved with ABR by using various types of canal electrode in order to enhance wave I. The signal can be transduced by an earphone mounted close to the ear, or by an insert earphone.

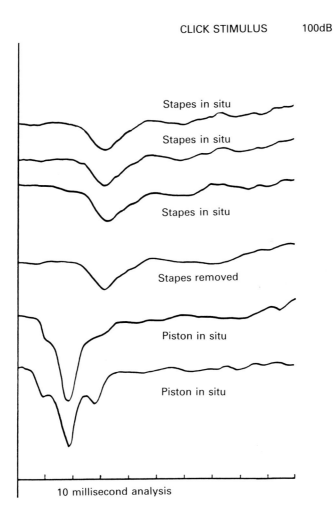

CLICK STIMULUS   100dB

Stapes in situ

Stapes in situ

Stapes in situ

Stapes removed

Piston in situ

Piston in situ

10 millisecond analysis

Fig. 17.1 Stapedectomy operative monitoring. Uncalibrated click stimulus ($\simeq100$ dB) (Reproduced with permission of Gibson W, unpublished).

STRATEGIES AND RESULTS DURING INTRA-OPERATIVE MONITORING

ECochG during middle ear surgery

By placing a silver ball electrode on the round window the ECochG response may be used to monitor stapedectomy surgery. Figure 17.1 shows three recordings taken prior to stapes removal. The response is delayed and low amplitude compared with normal values, indicating a marked degree of hearing loss. This is not unexpected as the normal air conduction route is not being used because the tympanum is reflected. However, the markedly improved and shorter latency responses which have a better morphology, obtained after the placement of the stapedial prosthesis shows clearly the improvement obtained by the operation. For a normally hearing subject a change in latency equal to the change obtained here would correspond to a 40–50 dB change in stimulus level.

ECochG monitoring during endolymphatic sac drainage operation

Preliminary results have shown that electrophysiologic change from abnormal toward normal SP/AP ratio can be achieved in endolymphatic sac drainage operations (Arenberg et al 1989). A significant reduction in SP/AP ratio was noted in 35% of cases. This intra-operative change is believed to indicate successful decompression of the hydropic endolymphatic fluid system.

The monitoring gives feedback to the surgeon if the hydropic labyrinth is successfully decompressed. Simple drainage may not achieve the decompression, and the change in SP may occur, for example, only on more proximal probing of the duct (Fig. 17.2).

If an abnormally enhanced SP cannot be significantly improved by any of the surgical manoeuvres, then the patient can avoid repeated sac-drainage operations, and can be offered vestibular nerve section.

Monitoring during the suboccipital posterior fossa approach in acoustic tumour surgery

Reversible ABR changes, including prolongation of intervals I–III and I–V or loss of all waves except I, together with retraction of the cerebellum and VIIIth nerve, can occur. Grundy et al (1982) have advised that intra-operative warning should be given if wave V latency increases by more than 1.5 ms. On the other hand, when the tumour is small, a gentle retraction does not produce discernible changes in ABR.

Relatively minor changes in CM, AP, and ABR may occur when drilling the IAM; and great changes, even sudden complete disappearance of the response, when dissecting the tumour in the meatus.

Recordings of CM and AP may suggest a direct vascular effect on the cochlea. It is difficult to separate CM from the electrical artefacts at high-

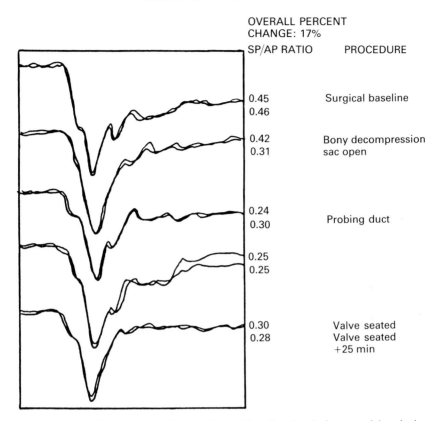

OVERALL PERCENT
CHANGE: 17%

SP/AP RATIO	PROCEDURE
0.45 0.46	Surgical baseline
0.42 0.31	Bony decompression sac open
0.24 0.30	Probing duct
0.25 0.25	
0.30 0.28	Valve seated Valve seated +25 min

Fig. 17.2 ECochG responses used to monitor cochlear function during an endolymphatic sac drainage operation (Reproduced with permission from Arenberg et al 1989).

stimulation levels, and one may have to rely on AP only. AP may disappear, but sometimes it gradually recovers when dissection is stopped. However, the AP may not recover, or sometimes it may gradually deteriorate because of developing changes in the small vessels (Fig. 17.3). Sometimes no potential apart from N1/I can be recorded prior to surgery, and then ECochG is the only guideline.

Relatively good preservation of wave I and slowly progressive deterioration of III and V components are more consistent with mechanical trauma than with vascular insufficiency. This could be due to desynchronization or blocked transmission. Even when wave V is absent at the end of the operation, it may return up to 2 weeks later. Reversible prolongation of V may be associated with the transient changes in hearing level.

Overall experience is that preservation of N1 and I is usually associated with some hearing preservation, but presence of wave I alone on ABR does not ensure that hearing will be saved. Wave I may be little affected when the tumour is dissected from the proximal part of the nerve, but wave I,

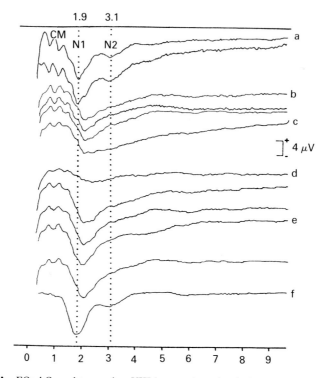

Fig. 17.3A ECochG used to monitor VIIIth nerve integrity during removal of a neuroma. (Reproduced with permission from Sabin 1987 Acta Neurochirurgica 85: 113).
a) before skin incision b) tumour manipulation c) drilling porus acousticus e) end of tumour dissection f) end of operation

together with hearing, can disappear a few weeks later. This can be due to the damage to the vascular supply. It has been observed that the major blood supply to the inner ear may remain intact at the operation, but it is possible that the loss of N1/I is due to disruption of its blood supply from the vasa vasorum following mechanical trauma.

It is difficult to evaluate to what extent the rapid feedback aids in preservation of hearing. However, the monitoring suggests various possible mechanisms of hearing dysfunction.

Intra-operative ABR in posterior fossa surgery

Introduction of the retractor and retraction of the cerebellum are an important step in adequate exposure of the surgical field, for example, in microvascular decompression for hemifacial spasm. The cochlear nerve, in particular, is vulnerable to retractor stretch and may produce changes on ABR. Boston et al (1987) observed systematic increase in latency I and in the interval I–III. Changes in peak I latency were most common, and usually showed substantial recovery at the end of the procedure. Changes in the

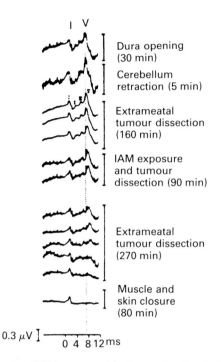

I   V

]   Dura opening
    (30 min)

]   Cerebellum
    retraction (5 min)

]   Extrameatal
    tumour dissection
    (160 min)

]   IAM exposure
    and tumour
    dissection (90 min)

]   Extrameatal
    tumour dissection
    (270 min)

]   Muscle and
    skin closure
    (80 min)

0.3 μV]   ———————
           0 4 8 12 ms

Fig. 17.3B   ABR to monitor VIIIth nerve and brainstem function during the removal of a neuroma. At the end of the operation the ABR shows wave I but no other peaks. This predicted that despite the VIIIth nerve integrity no functional hearing remained and this was confirmed by post operation, subjective and electrophysiological testing. (Reproduced with permission from Levin et al 1984 Annals of Otology, Rhinology and Laryngology 93: 117–120).

I–III interval were less common and smaller, but they were less likely to show recovery at the end of the operation. More radical change in ABR can occur, i.e. considerable prolongation of the latencies and loss of more rostral waves. In most cases, the surgeons were able to correct the retractor and modify their technique, which resulted in reduction of the latencies. In their study of 135 patients who had microvascular decompression for hemifacial spasm, Boston et al (1987) showed that in 15% of patients there was postoperative hearing deficit. In most cases, the hearing loss was mild (up to 20 dBHL) and generally transient, except in those cases in which ABR changes were radical or ABR was lost.

It has been suggested that ABR monitoring, and especially the knowledge that components III and IV remain intact, may help the surgeon in some difficult neurosurgical cases to decide to what extent to pursue tumours in the brainstem and towards the fourth ventricle (Bursick et al 1984).

18. Electrically evoked potentials in cochlear stimulation

CLINICAL PROBLEM

Population

Electrical stimulation of the cochlear nerve with unipolar and bipolar electrode systems has been devised as a cochlear prosthesis in which sounds are transformed into electrical stimuli through a processor. Clinical studies of multiple-electrode prostheses have shown that they provide significant help to postlingually deaf patients in understanding speech, especially when used in combination with lip-reading. About one half of such patients can understand some running speech without help from lip-reading (Clark et al 1987, Brown et al 1987). It has been estimated that there are about 3300 postlingually deaf adult subjects who may be considered for cochlear implant (Thornton 1986).

Tests for patient selection

Certain criteria are applied to the selection of patients for cochlear prosthesis implantation. However, some controversial issues have remained. A profound or total hearing loss should be recorded audiometrically, and the patient must be assessed with a hearing aid or tactile device to determine whether such an aid may be a substitute for a cochlear implant. The patient should have a zero score when tested with open sets of phonetically balanced words. Most centres select postlingually deaf adults, but in some centres children have been implanted. The correct psychiatric state, normal intelligence, and good medical condition are important for the successful management of these patients. Otological examination is necessary to exclude infection, and a CT scan of the middle ear cleft, inner ear, and CP angle is needed.

Subjective auditory threshold estimation of electrical cochlear stimulation and recording of evoked potentials in a profoundly deaf patient have been suggested as a method of pre-operative assessment of the viability of ganglion cells and neural fibres. The function of the implanted prosthesis can be objectively assessed by stimulating through the implanted electrode and evaluating the response. Evoked potentials similar to ABR and MLR can be recorded in man using extracochlear and intracochlear electrodes. These are known, respectively, as electrically evoked ABR (EABR) and electrically evoked MLR (EMLR).

METHODS OF ELECTRICALLY EVOKED POTENTIALS

Several methods of electrical stimulation have been described. Studies in experimental animals indicate that intracochlear stimulation from an electrode in the scala tympani produces better responses than does stimulation at the round window or the promontory when a large population of ganglion cells survive. In ears with almost no ganglion cells, the responses from the round window and the scala tympani are similar (Simmons et al 1987).

The needle electrode employed for ECochG can be used for stimulation by placing it on the promontory close to the round window. The current passes through another electrode attached to the ear lobe or mastoid. The transtympanic needle electrode often has an unfavourably high impedance.

A relatively small impedance can be achieved by using a platinum balled tip electrode placed into the round window through a small tympanotomy, and a second electrode placed on the promontory or the mastoid. The monopolar electrode used for cochlear implantation can successfully serve for pre-operative evaluation of auditory function with electrically evoked auditory potentials. Evoked potentials have been recorded by stimulating through the electrodes of an implanted extracochlear or intracochlear prosthesis (Fig. 18.1). Testing can be carried out in the operating room under anaesthesia or at a later date in the out-patient clinic. With general anaesthesia, the myogenic artefacts can be avoided on the EABR and EMLR recordings. Also, with extracochlear stimulation, higher stimulation levels can be attained without causing discomfort or pain.

Electrical stimuli with various duration and amplitude have been used. Diphasic rectangular electric pulses with duration of up to 200 μs or continuous square-wave stimuli have been used. With diphasic stimuli, more patients experience pain on stimulation. Currents of up to 1000 μA have been used for promontory, round window, and intracochlear stimulation (Smith & Simmons 1983, Game et al 1987, Black et al 1987, Rothera et al 1986). The behavioural threshold in μA of the current stimulus amplitude varies in deaf subjects. It is convenient to indicate the stimulus level in relative units in dB. The stimuli are presented at a rate of about 10/s and both EABR and EMLR can be recorded. The recording set-up is similar to acoustically evoked ABR and MLR. Problems caused by electrical artefacts during stimulation occur in early potentials of EABR. Electrical artefacts of the stimulus can be a problem, and artefact-suppression techniques are needed. This difficulty is absent for the later occurring EMLR.

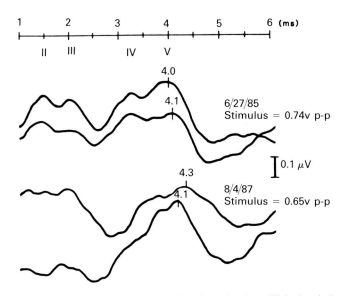

Fig. 18.1 ABR in response to electrical stimulation via an implant. With electrical stimulation that affects the nerve directly, the latencies are shorter than those obtained from acoustic stimulation (Upper trace: Initial result. Lower trace: two years postoperative). (After Miyamoto & Brown 1987.)

CHARACTERISTICS OF ELECTRICALLY EVOKED ABR AND MLR

EABR can be reliably reproduced. The EABR waveform is characterized by a shorter latency of the identifiable peaks when compared to the acoustically evoked ABR. The reduction in latency could be explained by the omission of the mechanical transmission and transduction processes.

Wave I is usually not identifiable and is overshadowed by electrical stimulus artefacts. Reproducible peaks within 5 ms can be identified and are thought to be consistent with waves III and wave V on ABR. At high intensities several other potentials can be noticed, including electromyographic activity from reflexive activation of the extra-ocular muscles at about 7 ms (Stypulkovski et al 1985).

Myogenic artefacts of the electrically evoked ABR were reported by Fifer & Novak (1987) when they stimulated the cochlea in a 34-month-old child, with a needle electrode placed against the round window niche, prior to inserting the cochlear implant. It was suggested that by stimulating with 100 μs duration pulses, a 1000 μA current produced stapedial muscle activity. At a threshold of 4000 μA with the needle electrode, a peak on the EABR occurred at 4.5 ms, and successively larger waves appeared with increase of the stimulus. When the muscles were paralysed, the larger waveforms disappeared; they were probably of myogenic origin. However, two peaks with latencies at 3.3 ms and 4.7 ms have maintained themselves with constant latency and amplitude, regardless of stimulation intensity, and these are thought to represent the EABR.

The amplitude of wave V varies and sometimes gets larger with increase of stimulus current. However, in deaf patients the limits of electrical stimulation have only a narrow dynamic range. An intracochlear implant stimulated EABR has been successfully recorded, and with an increase of the stimulus current from 500 to 1000 μA the amplitude of wave V, identified at about 5 ms, increases from about 150 to 350 nV (Game et al 1987). There is no definite change of latencies of the peaks, possibly due to well-synchronized neural response to electrical stimulation. Several investigators have recorded EABR using various stimulation techniques, and have identified wave III at 2.3–2.5 ms and wave V at 3.6–5.5 ms (Game et al 1987, Rothera et al 1986).

Changes in EABR in postimplantation patients using the 3M-House prosthesis showed that there are rapid changes at the electrode junction in the first 2 weeks followed by long-term stability (Waring et al 1987). Studying the EABR in the ossified cochleae after insertion of the intracochlear implant, one can apparently conclude that EABR threshold increases, corresponding to the degree of cochlear ossification.

Pre-operative clear EABR can be recorded only in a proportion of deaf patients. Electrical thresholds seem to be lower for round window stimulation compared to promontory stimulation, and it is more difficult to record by EABR employing a transtympanic needle technique. Analysing clinical results of postimplantation patients leads to the suggestion that EABR on its own is an inadequate predictor of surviving neurones and that additional tests are required.

Some information is available about other electrically evoked potentials. EMLRs in response to promontory stimulation were obtained in 19 out of 22 ears as a pre-operative evaluation for cochlear implantation (Kileny & Kemink 1987). The EMLR is characterized by peaks with latencies in the range of 20–30 ms, and the configuration closely resembles the acoustically evoked MLR. The EMLR thresholds correlate well with the behavioural thresholds, although the latter are lower. Further research into this potential is needed.

19. Current developments in ERA

In many areas electric response audiometry is an established and clinically useful tool. Its range of application is increasing into many different aspects.

DEVELOPMENTS IN RECORDING TECHNIQUES

As mentioned earlier, it is important in clinical practice to have a precise and accurate recording methodology. There have been significant moves towards standardization of the techniques involved and much of the optimization of the physical recording parameters has been completed and recommended standards have been published (Starr et al 1984).

Quality of the average response

Traditionally, evoked responses have been obtained by averaging a fixed number of sweeps. This means that in some cases test time has been wasted in obtaining sweeps which were not necessary whilst in other cases diagnostic decisions have been based upon poor waveforms for which more sweeps were needed. More flexible, adaptive procedures could be implemented if there was a rule for deciding how many sweeps are required to obtain a certain 'quality of response'. Quality estimation is based upon the signal/noise ratio and various methods of estimating this have been tried. It is important as this will permit a greater reliance to be placed on the diagnostic interpretation of good quality responses and, if the estimation is computed at the same time as the averaging process occurs, it would allow the operator to obtain just enough sweeps to give a certain quality of waveform. The resultant improvement in interpretation and saving in test time makes a significant advance to clinical practice.

The basis for most quality estimates is the measurement of the noise variance. Schimmel (1967) proposed the '± average' method to estimate this. For each pair of sweeps the second is subtracted from the first to cancel out the response component and leave only the noise. This is then stored in a separate memory area to that which contains the normal average. Wong & Bickford (1980) used this method as the basis of a quality estimator and Elberling & Don (1984) further developed the technique, making the estimator more robust against large amplitude, low frequency noise components. Several commercially available evoked response systems are beginning to implement such methods and this should improve the quality of clinical recordings.

Weighted averaging

Clinical experience indicates that the usual averaging procedure does not always perform well. Most clinicians with experience in this field will have come across cases in which increasing the number of sweeps can even lead to a less well-defined response. This occurs when the background noise is not 'stable'. Stationarity or 'stability' of the noise is fundamental to the application of averaging but as the patient changes his state of arousal so the noise can change. Hoke et al (1984) modelled this non-stationary behaviour and derived a weighted averaging technique which gave an improvement over normal averaging for such a process. Elberling & Wahlgreen (1985) developed this idea and, using Bayesian statistics, described an elegant and practical method of implementing weighted averaging. The averaging process is carried out in blocks of a relatively small number (approximately 250) sweeps. For each block the mean wave form and a noise variance are calculated and each block is weighted according to its noise variance. Thus blocks that come from noisier portions of the record contribute less to the final average than do the blocks that come from quiet sections of the record. In this way, short periods of high activity, or transients that contaminate the response, play very little part in the final average and this technique can give the same quality of response in a shorter time than normal averaging.

Further techniques

Research is continuing in many other areas and these are still remote from clinical practice and so will be mentioned only briefly.

The SQUID (Superconducting Quantum-Interference Device) is the device used to record the magnetic field produced by neural and myogenic activity. A conceivable advantage of magnetic as opposed to electrical recording lies in the possibility of directly estimating the generator site; the magnetic, tonotopic representation of the auditory slow vertex response has been reported by Pantev et al 1986).

Fundamental insight has been obtained from deconvolution techniques in which the normal click-evoked brainstem response is deconvolved with a unit response to give the compound impulse response of the brainstem generators. This mathematical exercise is useful because it is a means of effectively removing the changes to the response caused by peripheral hearing loss. Despite the advantages of this technique, its complexity has meant that it has not been applied as a routine clinical test.

Using three orthogonal electrode pairs, Williston et al (1981) recorded ABR data to produce a three dimensional representation in voltage/time space. Certain segments of this plot lie in a plane and the orientation of the plane can be altered by disorders of the auditory system. Further research is expected to refine the interpretation of the data and to investigate the effects of pathology.

Using a montage of 16 or more electrodes placed over the scalp, the evoked response amplitude at any instant can be mapped as isopotential lines. The potential at each electrode is used to interpolate the potentials at the points between the electrodes and, using colours to represent the potential value, a colour map of the evoked response distribution over the surface of the scalp can be generated. Such mapping techniques have been used both to gain fundamental knowledge and in clinical application (Morihisa et al 1983). More recently a technique of 'isochronic' mapping has been applied to the auditory brainstem responses (Thornton et al 1990). In this technique, lines of equal time, rather than isopotential lines, are plotted. The map therefore shows the latency of a particular peak in the response map over the scalp.

THRESHOLD ESTIMATION

The first clinical application of auditory evoked potentials was in threshold estimation. It is still used in this role and such applications have been discussed earlier.

Automated response detection

To make threshold estimation by evoked responses a truly objective process, automatic detection of the response is required. By eliminating the operator's subjective decisions about whether a response is present, evoked response techniques can be completely objective. A number of mathematical techniques for response detection and scoring have been applied to the slow cortical potential and more recently, such techniques have been applied to the ABR.

Some systems are based on the value of the correlation obtained between the test waveform and a template or 'standard waveform'. The template is sometimes obtained from the mean waveform given by many normally-hearing subjects (Elberling 1979), or the patient may be used as his own control and the template formed by his evoked response obtained at high stimulation levels. Depending on the value of the correlation coefficient, a decision is made as to whether a response is present or not.

Other correlation techniques used in threshold estimation involve calculating the value of the correlation coefficient between two responses obtained at the same stimulation level. Mason & Adams (1984) have reported such a system which uses both this correlation technique, together with an estimation of the variability of the background noise. A comparison of subjective and machine scoring of auditory brainstem responses in 75 patients has shown the acceptability of such methods.

Similar methods are being applied to neonatal screening. One system (Peters 1986) uses a nine-point template-matching detection algorithm together with binomial sampling of the 'noise' and the 'response plus noise'. Statistical calculations are based on these measures to provide a ratio of the probabilities that the event came from response plus noise or from the noise alone. The ratio of probabilities is known as a likelihood ratio and has to exceed a criterion value to register the decision that a response was present. In screening, such automated systems generally test at about 30 dB above normal threshold and simply indicate a pass or fail to the operator.

OBJECTIVE HEARING AID FITTING

Evoked responses have been used as objective threshold estimators to measure free field aided and unaided thresholds as part of the hearing aid prescription programme. Recently, a more direct approach has been tried. In order to fit a hearing aid to a very young child who can give no subjective responses, an estimate of the hearing threshold is required and an estimate of the upper end of the dynamic range of hearing is also needed. The loudness discomfort level (LDL) may be taken as an estimator of the upper end of the dynamic range and an objective method of estimating this has been developed (Thornton et al 1987). The relationship between the ABR wave V latency and subjective loudness was investigated to ascertain if objective estimation of LDL is possible. It was shown that the slope of the wave V latency input/output function did correlate to a high degree with the LDL. A predictive model of the LDL was derived and, for patients with hearing losses ranging from 35–80 dB HTL in the frequency range 2–4 kHz, the LDL was predicted to within ±8 dB for 95% of the sample.

Work is currently proceeding to use this as a means of objectively fitting hearing aids to very young children. The basic concept is that the threshold will be estimated in the normal way using ABR and the LDL estimated with this technique. During the procedure, the sound pressure levels in the ear canal will be monitored with a probe microphone using a 1 mm flexible probe tube. A hearing aid may then be fitted and the sound pressure levels monitored again with the same probe microphone. The hearing aid can then be adjusted so that conversation level sounds are above threshold and loud sounds do not exceed the LDL as monitored within the patient's ear canal with the probe microphone.

ABR IN MÉNIÈRE'S SYNDROME

As previously mentioned (p. 110), it is possible to use the ABR to estimate the speed of the wave motion along the basilar membrane. The travelling wave velocity (TWV) has been estimated using derived response (Parker & Thornton 1978). Recently this technique has been applied to the diagnosis of endolymphatic hydrops under the following experimental hypothesis. If the pressure in the scala media is increased then the stiffness of the basilar membrane will also be increased and hence increase the speed of the travelling wave.

It has been shown (Thornton & Farrell 1989) that the TWV measures at high frequencies are increased for Ménière's patients. It was also demonstrated that this increase was not due to the pathologically broadened tuning curves in these patients. The technique was then clinically verified by monitoring patients undergoing a glycerol dehydration procedure. For all patients who showed a positive audiometric change, the travelling wave velocity moved from abnormal towards normal values. A short, clinical version of this test which takes only 15–30 minutes, has been devised and the additional hardware to enable this method to be carried out with standard evoked response equipment is undergoing clinical trials at three centres. A diagnostic test which is specific to endolymphatic hydrops and which can be used to monitor the effects of drugs and to compare drugs, will clearly be useful both in the initial assessment and in the management of patients.

References

Abramovich S J 1987 Auditory brainstem response and computed tomography in acoustic tumour investigations. Journal of Laryngology and Otology 101: 334–345

Abramovich S J 1988 Effect of age and cochlear hearing loss on the auditory brainstem potentials. Clinical Otolaryngology 13: 74

Abramovich S J, Billings R 1981 Cochlear and brainstem auditory evoked potential recording in patients with unilateral sensorineural hearing loss. Journal of Laryngology and Otology 95: 925–950

Abramovich S J, Billings R 1981 Transtympanic electrocochleography and brainstem auditory evoked potentials in patients with unilateral sensorineural hearing loss. ERA Newsletter (VIIth symposium): p M1

Abramovich S J, Gregory S, Slemick M, Stewart A 1979 Hearing loss in very low birthweight infants treated with neonatal intensive care. Archives of Disease in Childhood 54: 421–426

Abramovich S J, Hyde M L, Riko K, Alberti P W 1987 Early detection of hearing loss in high risk children using brainstem electrical response audiometry. Journal of Laryngology and Otology 101: 120–126

Abramovich S J, Prasher D K 1986 Electrocochleograpy and brainstem potentials in Ramsay Hunt syndrome. Archives of Otolaryngology 112: 925–928

Adrian E D 1931 The microphonic action of the cochlea in relation to theories of hearing. In: Report of a discussion of audition. Physical Society of London: 5–9

Alberti P W, Hyde M L, Riko K, Corbin H, Abramovich S J 1983 An evaluation of BERA for hearing screening in high-risk neonates. Laryngoscope 93: 1115–1121

Allen A R, Starr A 1978 Auditory brainstem potentials in monkeys (M. mulatta) and man. Electroencephalography and Clinical Neurophysiology 45: 53–63

Andreev A M, Arapova A A, Gersuni S V 1939 On electrical potentials in the human cochlea. Journal of Physiology (London) 26: 205–212

Antoli-Candela F, Kiang N Y-S 1978 Unit activity underlying the N1 potential. In: Naunton R F, Fernandez C (eds) Evoked electrical activity in the auditory nervous system. Academic Press, New York

Aran J-M 1971 The electrocochleogram; recent results in children and in some pathological cases. Archives für Klinische und experimentelle Ohres-Nases und Kehlkopfheilkunde 198: 128–141

Aran J-M 1973 Clinical measures of eighth nerve function. Advances in Otorhinolaryngology (Basel) 20: 374–394

Aran J-M, Charlet de Sauvage R 1976 Clinical value of cochlear microphonic recordings. In: Ruben R J, Elberling C, Salomon G (eds) Electrocochleography. University Park Press, Baltimore, Md., pp. 55–65

Arenberg I K, Gibson W P R, Bohlen K H 1989 Improvements in audiometric and electrophysiologic parameters following nondestructive inner ear surgery utilizing a valved shunt for hydrops and Ménière's disease. In: Nadol J B (ed) Second International Symposium on Ménière's Disease. Kugler & Ghedini Publications, Amsterdam pp 545–561

Barajas J J 1982 Evaluation of ipsilateral and contralateral brainstem auditory evoked potentials in multiple sclerosis patients. Journal of Neurological Sciences 54: 69–78

Barrs D M, Brackmann D E, Olson J E, House W F 1985 Changing concepts of acoustic neuroma diagnosis. Archives of Otolaryngology 111: 17–21

Bauch C D, Rose D E, Harner S G 1982 Auditory brainstem response results from 255 patients with suspected retrocochlear involvement. Ear and Hearing 3: 83–86

Bauer H J 1980 IMAB-enquete concerning the diagnostic criteria for MS. In: Bauer H J, Poser S, Ritter G (eds) Progress in multiple sclerosis research. Springer, Berlin, pp 555–563

Beagley H A, Fateen A M, Gordon A G 1972 Clinical experience of evoked response and subjective auditory thresholds. Sound 6: 8–13

Beagley H A, Kellogg S E 1969 A comparison of evoked response and subjective auditory thresholds. International Audiology 8: 345–353

Beagley H A, Sheldrake J B 1978 Differences in brainstem response latency with age and sex. British Journal of Audiology 12: 69–77

Békésy G Von 1951 D-C potentials and energy balance of the cochlear partition. Journal of the Acoustic Society of America 23: 576 82

Békésy G Von 1960 Experiments in hearing. Trans. Wever E G. McGraw-Hill, New York

Bell I E, Thornton A R D 1988 Measures for the optimum estimation of audiometric thresholds from the auditory brainstem response potentials. British Journal of Audiology 22: 21–27

Bellman S, Barnard S, Beagley H A 1984 A nine-year review of 841 children tested by transtympanic electrocochleography. Journal of Laryngology and Otology 98: 1–9

Ben-David J, Gertner R, Podoshin L, Fradis M, Pratt H, Rabina A 1986 Auditory brainstem evoked potentials in patients suffering from peripheral facial nerve palsy and diabetes mellitus. Journal of Laryngology and Otology 100: 629–633

Bennett M J 1979 Trials with the auditory response cradle I – neonatal responses to auditory stimuli. British Journal of Audiology 13: 125–134

Bennett M J 1980 Trials with the auditory response cradle II – the neonatal respiratory response to an auditory stimulus. British Journal of Audiology 14: 1–6

Bennett M J 1980 Trials with the auditory response cradle III – head turns and startles as auditory responses in the neonate. British Journal of Audiology 14: 122–131

Berger H 1929 Über das Elektrencephalogramm des Menschen. Archiv für Psychiatrie und Nervenkrankheiten 87: 527–570

Bergholtz L M, Arlinger S D, Kylen P, Jerlvall L B 1977 Electrocochleography used as a clinical hearing test in difficult-to-test children. Acta Otolaryngologica 84: 385–392

Bhattacharya J, Bennett M J, Tucker S M 1984 Long term follow-up of newborns tested with the auditory response cradle. Archives of Disease in Childhood 59: 504–511

Bickford R G, Jacobson J L, Cody D T R 1964 Nature of averaged evoked potentials to sound and other stimuli in man. Annals of New York Academy of Science 112: 204–223

Black F O, Lilly D J, Fowler L P, Stypulkowski P H 1987 Surgical evaluation of candidates for cochlear implants. Annals of Otology, Rhinology and Laryngology (suppl. 128) 96: 96–99

Booth J P 1980 Ménière's disease: the selection and assessment of patients for surgery using electrocochleography. Annals of the Royal College of Surgeons of England 62: 415–425

Borg E, Lofqvist L 1982 Auditory brainstem response to rarefaction and condensation clicks in normal and abnormal ears. Scandinavian Audiology 11: 227–235

Boston J R, Ainslie P J 1980 Effects of analog and digital filtering on brainstem auditory evoked potentials. Electroencephalography and Clinical Neurophysiology 48: 361–364

Boston J R, Deneault L, Kronk L, Jannetta P 1987 Continuous monitoring of BAEP during retromastoid craniotomies. International Electric Response Audiometry Study Group X Biennial Symposium (Charlottesville,). ERA Newsletter 19: 123

Brackmann D E, Selters W A 1976 Electrocochleography in Ménière's disease and acoustic neuromas. In: Ruben R J, Elberling C, Salomon G, (eds) Electrocochleography. University Park Press, Baltimore, Md., pp 315–329

Bradford B C, Baudin J, Conway M J et al 1985 Identification of sensory neural hearing loss in very preterm infants by brainstem auditory evoked potentials. Archives of Disease in Childhood 60: 105–109

Brewer C C, Resnick D M 1984 The value of BAEP in assessment of the comatose patient. In: Nodar R H, Barber C (eds) Evoked potentials II. Butterworth, Boston, Mass., pp 578–581

Brinkman R D, Scherg M 1979 Human auditory on- and off-potentials of the brainstem. Scandinavian Audiology 3: 27–32

Brown A M, Dowell R C, Clark G M 1987 Clinical results for postlingually deaf patients implanted with multichannel cochlear prostheses. Annals of Otology, Rhinology and Laryngology (suppl. 128) 96: 127–128

Buchwald J S 1983 Generators. In: Moore E J (ed) Bases of auditory brain-stem potential in nervous system. Academic Press, New York

Buchwald J S, Hinman C, Norman R J et al 1981 Middle- and long-latency auditory evoked responses recorded from the vertex of normal and chronically-lesioned cats. Brain Research 205: 91–109

Buchwald J S, Huang C M 1975 Far-field acoustic response: Origins in the cat. Science 189: 382–384

Burian K, Gestring G F 1971 Discrepancies between subjective and objective acoustic thresholds. Archiv für Klinische und experimentelle Ohren-Nasen-und Kehlkopfheilkunde 198: 73–82

Burkard R, Hecox K 1983 The effect of broadband noise on the human brainstem auditory response II: Frequency specificity. Journal of the Acoustic Society of America 74: 1214–1223

Bursick D M, Vries J K, Sclabassi R J, Guthkelch A N 1984 Intraoperative brainstem evoked potentials as an adjunct to posterior fossa surgery in children. In: Nodar R H, Barber C (eds) Evoked potentials II (The Second International Evoked Potential Symposium). Butterworth, Boston, Mass., pp 565–571

Cashman M Z, Rossman R N 1983 Diagnostic features of the auditory brainstem response in identifying cerebellopontine angle tumours. Scandinavian Audiology 12: 35–42

Catlin F I 1978 Etiology and pathology of hearing loss in children. In: Martin F N (ed) Pediatric Audiology. Prentice-Hall, Englewood Cliffs, N.J. pp 3–34

Charlet de Sauvage R, Aran J-M 1976 Clinical value of adaptation measurements in electrocochleography. In: Ruben J R, Elberling C, Salomon G (eds) Electrocochleography. University Park Press, Baltimore, Md., pp 169–182

Chiappa K H 1983 Evoked potentials in clinical medicine: pattern shift visual, brainstem auditory and short latency somatosensory: techniques, correlations and interpretations. Raven Press, New York

Chiappa K H, Gladstone K J, Joung R R 1979 Brainstem auditory evoked responses. Studies of waveform variations in 50 normal human subjects. Archives of Neurology 36: 81–87

Chiappa K H, Ropper A H 1982 Evoked potentials in clinical medicine: Part 1. New England Journal of Medicine 306: 1140–1210

Clark G M, Blamey P J, Brown A M et al 1987 The University of Melbourne – Nucleus multi-electrode cochlear implant. Advances in Otorhinolaryngology 38: 1–181

Clemis J D, Mastricola P G 1976 Special audiometric test battery in 121 proved acoustic tumors. Archives of Otolaryngology 102: 654–656

Clemis J D, McGee T 1979 Brainstem electric response audiometry in differential diagnosis of acoustic tumours. Laryngoscope 84: 31–42

Coats A C 1974 On electrocochleographic electrode design. Journal of the Acoustic Society of America 56: 708–711

Coats A C 1978 Human auditory nerve action potentials and brainstem evoked responses. Latency-intensity functions in detection of cochlear and retrocochlear abnormality. Archives of Otolaryngology 104: 709

Coats A C 1986 Normal summating potential recorded from the external ear canal. Archives of Otolaryngology – Head and Neck Surgery 112: 759–768

Coats A C, Alford B P 1981 Ménière's disease and summating potential III: Effect of glycerol administration. Archives of Otolaryngology 107: 469–473

Coats A C, Kidder H R 1930 Earspeaker coupling effects on auditory action potential and brainstem response. Archives of Otolaryngology 106: 339–344

Coats A C, Martin J L 1977 Human auditory nerve action potentials and brainstem evoked responses. Archives of Otolaryngology 103: 605–622

Cooper R, Osselton J W, Shaw J C 1974 EEG technology. Butterworth, London

Crawford A C, Fettiplace R 1985 The mechanical properties of ciliary bundles of turtle cochlear hair cells. Journal of Physiology 364: 359–379

Crosby E, Humphrey T, Lauer E 1962 Correlative anatomy of the nervous system. Macmillan, New York

Crowley D E, Davis H, Beagley H 1976 Clinical use of electrocochleography: A preliminary report. In: Ruben R J, Elberling C, Salomon C (eds) Electrocochleography. University Park Press, Baltimore, Md., pp 287–294

Cullen J K, Ellis M S, Berlin C I, Lowsteau R J 1972 Human acoustic nerve action potential recordings from the tympanic membrane without anaesthesia. Acta Otolaryngologica (Stockholm) 74: 15–22

Dallos P 1973 Cochlear potentials and cochlear mechanics. In: Moller A (ed) Basic mechanisms of hearing. Academic Press, New York, pp 335–376

Dallos P 1975 Electrical correlates of mechanical events in the cochlea. Audiology 14: 408–418

Dallos P 1976 Cochlear receptor potentials. In: Ruben R J, Elberling C, Salomon G (eds) Electrocochleography. University Park Press, Baltimore, Md., pp 5–21

Dallos P 1985 Response characteristics of mammalian cochlear hair cells. Journal of Neurosciences 5: 1591–1608

Dallos P, Billone M, Durrant J D, Wang C-Y, Raynor S 1972 Cochlea inner and outer hair cells: Functional differences. Science 177: 356–358

Dallos P, Schoeny Z G, Cheatham M A 1972 Cochlear summating potentials: Descriptive aspects. Acta Otolaryngologica (suppl.) 302: 46

Dallos P, Wang C-Y 1974 Bioelectric correlates of kanamycin intoxication. Audiology 13: 277–287

Dauman R, Aran J-M, Charlet de Sauvage R, Portmann M 1988 Clinical significance of the summating potential in Ménière's disease. American Journal of Otology 9: 31–38

Dauman R, Aran J-M, Portmann M 1986 Summating potential and water balance in Ménière's disease. Annals of Otology, Rhinology and Laryngology 95: 389–395

Davies A 1984 Detecting hearing-impairment in neonates – the statistical decision criterion for the auditory response cradle. British Journal of Audiology 18: 163–168

Davis H 1965 A model for transducer action in the cochlea. Cold Spring Harbor Symposium in Quantitative Biology 30: 181–189

Davis H 1976 Principles of electric response audiometry. Annals of Otology, Rhinology, and Laryngology (suppl. 28) 85: 1–96

Davis H 1981 Electric response audiology: Past, present and future. Ear and hearing 2: 5–8

Davis H 1984 Auditory evoked potentials. In: Nodar R H, Barber C (eds) Evoked potentials II. Butterworth, Boston, Mass., pp 17–24

Davis H, Darbyshire A, Lurie M, Saul L 1934 The electric response of the cochlea. American Journal of Physiology 107: 317–332

Davis H, Deatherage B H, Rosenblut B, Fernandez C, Kimura R, Smith A 1958 Modification of cochlear potentials produced by streptomycin poisoning and by extensive venous obstruction. Laryngoscope 68: 596–627

Davis H, Fernandez C, McAuliffe D R 1950 The excitatory process in the cochlea. Proceedings of the National Academy of Science (USA) 36: 580–587

Davis H, Hirsh S K 1979 A slow brainstem response for low frequency audiometry. Audiometry 18: 445–461

Davis H, Tasaki T, Goldstein R 1952 The peripheral origin of activity, with reference to the ear. Cold Spring Harbor Symposium on Quantitative Biology 17: 143–154

Davis H, Zerlin S 1966 Acoustic relations of the human vertex potential. Journal of the Acoustic Society of America 39: 109–116

Davis P A 1939 Effects of acoustic stimuli on the waking human brain. Journal of Neurophysiology 2: 494

Dawson G D 1951 A summation technique for detecting small signals in a large irregular background. Journal of Physiology (London) 115: 2

Djupesland G, Flottorp G, Modalsli B, Tvete O, Sortland O 1981 Acoustic brainstem response in diagnosis of acoustic neuroma. Scandinavian Audiology (suppl.) 13: 109–112

Dohlmann C F 1983 Histopathology and pathophysiology of Ménière's disease. In: Oosterveld W J (ed) Ménière's disease: a comprehensive appraisal. John Wiley, New York, pp 55–90

Don M, Allen A R, Starr A 1977 Effect of click rate on the latency of auditory brainstem responses in humans. Annals of Otology, Rhinology and Laryngology 86: 186–196

Don M, Eggermont J J 1978 Analysis of the click-evoked brainstem potentials in man using high-pass noise masking. Journal of the Acoustic Society of America 63: 1084–1092

Douek E, Gibson W P R, Humphries K N 1973 The crossed acoustic response. Journal of Laryngology and Otology 87: 711–726

Doyle D J, Hyde M L 1981 Analogue and digital filtering of auditory brainstem potentials. Scandinavian Audiology 10: 81–89

Duncan P G, Sanders R A, McCullough D W 1979 Preservation of auditory-evoked brainstem responses in anaesthetised children. Canadian Anaesthesiology Society Journal 26: 492–495

Durrant J D, Lovrinic J H 1984 Bases of hearing science. 2nd edn. Williams, Baltimore, Md.

Eggermont J J 1976 Summating potentials in electrocochleography: Relation to hearing disorders. In: Ruben R J, Elberling C, Salomon G (eds) Electrocochleography. University Park Press, Baltimore, Md., pp 67–87

Eggermont J J 1977 Compound action potential tuning curves in normal and pathological human ears. Journal of the Acoustic Society of America 62: 1247–1251

Eggermont J J 1979 Human electrocochleography. In: Beagley H A (ed) Auditory investigation: The scientific and technological basis. Clarendon Press, Oxford

Eggermont J J 1982 The inadequacy of click-evoked auditory brainstem responses in audiological applications. Annals of the New York Academy of Science 388: 707–709

Eggermont J J, Don M 1980 Analysis of the click-evoked brainstem potentials in humans using high-pass noise masking II: Effects of click intensity. Journal of the Acoustic Society of America 68: 1671–1675

Eggermont J J, Don M, Brackmann D E 1980 Electrocochleography and auditory brainstem electric responses in patients with pontine angle tumours. Annals of Otology, Rhinology and Laryngology (suppl. 75) 89: 1–19

Eggermont J J, Odenthal D W 1974 Action potentials and summating potentials in the normal human cochlea. Acta Otolaryngologica. (suppl.) 316: 39–61

Eggermont J J, Odenthal D W 1977 Potentialities of clinical electrocochleography. Clinical Otolaryngology 2: 275–286

Eggermont J J, Spoor A, Odenthal D W 1976 Frequency specificity of tone-burst electrocochleography. In: Ruben J R, Elberling C, Salomon G (eds) Electrocochleography. University Park Press, Baltimore, Md., pp 215–246

Elbering C 1974 Action potentials along the cochlear partition recorded from the ear canal in man. Scandinavian Audiology 3: 13–19

Elberling C 1976 Simulation of cochlear action potentials recorded from the ear canal in man. In: Ruben J R, Elberling C, Salomon G (eds) Electrocochleography. University Park Press, Baltimore, Md., pp 151–168

Elberling, C 1979 Auditory electrophysiology. Use of templates and cross-correlation functions in the analysis of brainstem potentials. Scandinavian Audiology 8: 187–190

Elberling C, Donn M 1984 Quality estimation of averaged auditory brainstem responses. Scandinavian Audiology 13: 187–197

Elberling C, Salomon G 1971 Electrical potentials from the inner ear in man in response to transient sounds generated in a closed acoustic system. Revue de Laryngologie (Bordeaux) 92: 691–707

Elberling C, Wahlgreen O 1985 Estimation of auditory brainstem response, ABR, by means of Bayesian inference. Scandinavian Audiology 14: 89–96

Eldredge D H 1974 Inner ear–cochlear mechanics and cochlear potentials. In: Keidel W D, Neff W D (eds) Handbook of sensory, physiology: Auditory system. Springer-Verlag, Berlin, pp 549–584

Engel R 1969 Calibrated pure tone audiogram in normal neonates based on evoked electroencephalographic responses. Neuropadiatrie 1: 149

Evans E F 1975 Normal and abnormal functioning of the cochlear nerve. In: Bench R J, Pye A, Pye J E (eds) Sound reception in mammals. Academic Press, London pp 133–165

Feinmesser M, Tell L 1976 Methods for detecting hearing impairment in infancy and early childhood. In: Mencher G T (ed) Early identification of hearing loss. Karger, Basel, pp 102–113

Feinmesser M, Tell L, Levy H 1982 Follow-up of 40 000 infants screened for hearing defects. Audiology 21: 197–203

Ferraro J A, Arenberg I K, Hassanein R S 1985 Electrocochleography and symptoms of inner ear dysfunction. Archives of Otolaryngology 111: 71–74

Fifer R, Novak M 1987 Myogenic influences of the electrically evoked ABR. International Electric Response Audiometry Study Group x Biennial Symposium (Charlottesville, V). ERA Newsletter 19: 187

Finitzo-Hieber T, Friel-Patti S 1985 Conductive hearing loss and ABR. In: Jacobson J T (ed) The auditory brainstem response. College-Hill Press, San Diego, Calif., pp 113–131

Fraser J G, Conway M J, Keen M H, Hazell J W P 1978 The postauricular myogenic response: A new instrument which simplifies its detection by machine scoring. Journal of Laryngology and Otology 92: 293–303

Fria T J, Sabo D L 1980 Auditory brainstem responses in children with otitis media with effusion. Annals of Otology, Rhinology and Laryngology 68: 200–206

Fria T J, Saad M M, Doyle W J, Cantekin E I 1984 Slow negative evoked potentials in the rhesus monkey (*Macaca mulatta*): Myogenic versus neurogenic influences. Electroencephalography and Clinical Neurophysiology 59: 81

Friedmann I 1974 *Herpes zoster* oticus. In: Friedmann I Pathology of the ear. Blackwell, Boston, Mass., pp 442–448

Friedmann I 1974 Pathology of the ear. Blackwell, Boston, Mass.

Frishkopf L S, DeRosier D J 1983 Mechanical tuning of free-standing stereociliary bundles and frequency analysis in the alligator lizard cochlea. Hearing Research 12: 393–404

Fromm B, Nylen C O, Zotterman Y 1935 Studies in the mechanism of the Wever–Bray effect. Acta Otolaryngologica (Stockholm) 22: 477–486

Frye-Osier H A, Goldstein R, Hirsch J E, Waber K 1982 Early and middle AER components to clicks as response indices for neonatal hearing screening. Annals of Otology, Rhinology and Laryngology 19: 272–276

Gacek R R, Rasmussen G L 1961 Fiber analysis of the statoacoustic nerve of guinea pig, cat and monkey. Anatomical Record 139: 455–463

Galambos R 1958 Neural mechanism of audition. Laryngoscope 68: 388–403

Galambos R 1978 Use of auditory brainstem response (ABR) in infant hearing testing. In: Gerber S E, Mencher G T (eds) Early diagnosis of hearing loss. Grune & Stratton, New York

Galambos R G, Despland P A 1980 The auditory brainstem response (ABR) evaluates risk factors for hearing loss in newborns. Pediatric Research 14: 159–163

Galambos R, Hicks G, Wilson M J 1982 Hearing loss in graduates of tertiary intensive care nursery. Ear and Hearing 3: 87–90

Galambos R, Makeing S, Talmachoff P J 1981 A 40-Hz auditory potential recorded from the human scalp. Proceedings of the National Academy cf Science (USA) 78: 2643–2647

Game C J A, Gibson W P R, Pauka C K 1987 Electrically evoked brainstem auditory potentials. Annals of Otology, Rhinology and Laryngology (suppl. 128) 96: 94–95

Geddes L A, Baker L E 1967 In: Geddes L A (ed) Electrodes and the measurement of bioelectric events. Wiley, New York

Geisler C D, Frishkopf L S, Rosenblith W A 1958 Extracranial responses to acoustic clicks in man. Science 128: 1210–1211

Geisler C D, Sinex D G 1980 Responses of primary auditory fiber to combined noise and tonal stimuli. Hearing Research 3: 317–334

Gersuni G V, Andreev A M, Arapova A A 1937 Proceedings of the Academy of Science SSSR 16: 429

Gerull G, Mrowinski D 1984 Brainstem potentials evoked by binaural click stimuli with differences in interaural time and intensity. Audiology 23: 265–276

Gibson W P R 1978 Essentials of clinical electric response audiometry. Churchill Livingstone, Edinburgh

Gibson W P R, Beagley H A 1976 Electrocochleography in diagnosis of acoustic neuroma. Journal of Laryngology and Otology 90: 127–140

Gibson W P R, Prasher D K, Kilkenny G P G 1983 Diagnostic significance of transtympanic electrocochleography in Meniere's disease. Annals of Otology, Rhinology and Laryngology 92: 155–159

Gibson W P R, Ramsden R T, Moffat D A 1977 Clinical electrocochleography in diagnosis and management of Meniere's disease. Audiology 16: 389–401

Goff W R, Williamson P O, Van Gilder J C, Allison T, Fisher T C 1980 Neural origins of long latency evoked cortical potentials recorded from the depth and from the cortical surfaces of the brain in man. In: Desmedt J (ed) Progress in clinical neurophysiology vol 7: Clinical uses of cerebral, brainstem and spinal somatosensory evoked potentials. Karger, Basel

Goldstein R, Rodman L B 1967 Early components of averaged evoked responses to rapidly repeated auditory stimuli. Journal of Speech and Hearing Research 10: 697–705

Goodin D S, Squires K C, Starr A 1978 Long latency event-related components of the auditory evoked potentials in dementia. Brain 101: 635–648

Gordon E, Kraiuhin C, Stanfield P et al 1986 The prediction of normal P3 latency and the diagnosis of dementia. Neuropsychologia 24: 823–830

Graham J M 1981 Tinnitus and deafness of sudden onset: Electrocochleographic findings in 100 patients. Journal of Laryngology and Otology (suppl. 4) pp 111–116

Grundy B L, Jannetta P J, Procopio P T, Lina A, Boston R, Doyle E 1982 Intraoperative monitoring of brain-stem auditory evoked potentials. Journal of Neurosurgery 57: 674–681

Grundy B L, Lina A, Procopio P T, Jannetta P J 1981 Reversible evoked potential changes with retraction of the eighth cranial nerve. Anaesthesia and Analgesia 60: 835–838

Gutnick H N, Goldstein R 1978 Effect of contralateral noise on the middle components of the averaged electroencephalic response. Journal of Speech and Hearing Research 21: 613–624

Halgren E, Squires N K, Wilson C L, Rohrbaugh J W, Babb T L, Crandall P H 1980 Endogenous potentials generated in the human hippocampal formation and amygdala by infrequent effects. Science 210: 803–805

Hall J W, Mackey-Hargadine J R, Allen S J 1985 Monitoring neurologic status of comatose patients in the intensive care unit. In: Jacobson J T (ed) The auditory brainstem response. College-Hill Press, San Diego, Calif., pp 252–286

Hallpike C S, Cairns H 1938 Observations on the pathology of Ménière's syndrome. Journal of Laryngology and Otology 53: 625–655

Harker L A, Hosick E C, Voots R J, Mendel M I 1977 Influence of succinylcholine on middle component auditory evoked potentials. Archives of Otolaryngology 103: 133–137

Harrison R V 1987 Auditory science tutorial III: The role of the ascending pathways. Journal of Otolaryngology, 16: 80–88

Harrison R V, Aran J-M 1982 Electrocochleographic measures of frequency selectivity in human deafness. British Journal of Audiology 16: 179–188

Hashimoto I 1982 Auditory evoked potentials from the human midbrain: Slow brainstem responses. Electroencephalography and Clinical Neurophysiology 50: 254

Hashimoto I, Ishiyama Y, Tozuka G 1979 Bilaterally recorded brainstem auditory evoked responses. Archives of Neurology 36: 161–167

Hashimoto I, Ishiyama Y, Yoshimoto T, Nemoto S 1981 Brainstem auditory evoked potentials recorded directly from human brain-stem and thalamus. Brain 104: 841–859

Hayes D, Jerger J 1982 Auditory brainstem response to tone-pips: Results in normal and hearing-impaired subjects. Scandinavian Audiology 11: 133–142

Hecox K 1985 Neurologic applications of the auditory brainstem response to the paediatric age group. In: Jacobson J T (ed) The auditory brainstem response. College-Hill Press, San Diego, Calif., pp 288–295

Hecox K, Burkhard R 1982 Developmental dependancies of the human brainstem auditory evoked response. Annals of the New York Academy of Sciences 388: 338–556

Hecox K E, Cone B, Blaw M E 1931 Brainstem auditory evoked responses in the diagnosis of pediatric neurologic diseases. Neurology 31: 832–840

Hesse G 1987 Pre-surgical evaluation in cochlear-implants: Summating potentials with complete inner-ear deafness. International Electric Response Audiometry Study Group X Biennial Symposium. ERA Newsletter 19: 184

Hillyard S A 1984 Cognitive functions and event-related brain potentials. In: Nodar R H, Barber C (eds) Evoked potentials II (The Second International Evoked Potentials Symposium). Butterworth, Boston, Mass., pp 51–62

Hillyard S A, Picton T W 1979 Event-related brain potentials and selective information processing in man. In: Desmedt J E (ed) Progress in clinical neurophysiology vol 6: Cognitive components in cerebral event-related potentials and selective attention. Karger, Basel, pp 1–52

Hoke M 1976 Cochlear microphonics in man and its probable importance in objective audiometry. In: Rubin R J, Elberling C, Salomon G (eds) Electrocochleography. University Park Press, Baltimore, Md., pp 41–54

Hoke M, Ross B, Wickesberg R, Lutkenhoner B 1984 Weighted averaging – theory and application to electric response audiometry. Electroencephalopathy and Clinical Neurophysiology 57: 484–489

Horiuchi K 1976 Auditory middle latency response. Journal of Otolaryngology of Japan 79: 1549–1558

House W F, Luetje C M 1979 Acoustic tumors vol I: Diagnosis. University Park Press, Baltimore, Md.

Huang C M 1980 A comparative study of the brainstem auditory response in mammals. Brain Research 184: 215–219

Huang C M, Buchwald J S 1978 Factors that affect the amplitudes and latencies of the vertex short latency acoustic responses in the cat. Electroencephalography and Clinical Neurophysiology 44: 179–186

Hudspeth A J 1985 The cellular basis of hearing: the biophysics of hair cells. Science 230: 745–752

Hutton J N T 1981 Sedation and anaesthesia. In: Beagley H A (ed) Audiology and audiological medicine. Oxford University Press, Oxford, vol 2, pp 809–815

Hyde M L 1985 The effect of cochlear lesions on the ABR. In: Jacobson J T (ed) The auditory brainstem response. College-Hill Press, San Diego, Calif., pp 133–146

Hyde M L 1985 Frequency-specific BERA in infants. Journal of Otolaryngology (suppl. 14) 14: 19–27

Hyde M, Alberti P, Matsumoto N, Yao-Li Li 1986 Auditory evoked potentials in audiometric assessment of compensation and medicolegal patients. Annals of Otology, Rhinology and Laryngology 95: 514–519

Hyde M L, Blair R L 1981 The auditory brain-stem response in neuro-otology: Perspective and problems. Journal of Otolaryngology 10: 117–125

Hyde M L, Stephens S D G, Thornton A R D 1976 Stimulus repetition rate and the early brainstem responses. British Journal of Audiology 10: 41–50

Jacobson G P, Means E D, Dhib-Jalbut S 1986 Delay in the absolute latency of auditory brainstem response (ABR) component P1 in acute inflammatory demyelinating disease. Scandinavian Audiology 15: 121–124

Jacobson J T, Hyde M 1984 An introduction to auditory evoked potentials. In: Katz J (ed) Handbook of clinical audiology. Williams, Baltimore, Md.

Jacobson J T, Seitz M R, Mencher G, Parrott V F 1981 Auditory brainstem response: A contribution to infant assessment and management. In: Mencher G, Gerber S (eds) Early management of hearing loss. Grune & Stratton, New York

Jacobson J T, Morehouse C R, Johnson M J 1982 Strategies for infant auditory brainstem response assessment. Ear and Hearing 3: 263–270

Jasper H H 1958 Report of the committee on methods of clinical examination in electroencephalography. Electroencephalography and Clinical Neurophysiology 10: 370

Javel E, Mouney D F, McGee J, Walsh E J 1982 Auditory brainstem responses during systemic infusion of lidocaine. Archives of Otolaryngology 108: 71–76

Jerger J, Hall J 1980 Effects of age and sex on the auditory brainstem response. Archives of Otolaryngology 106: 382–391

Jerger J, Mauldin L 1978 Prediction of sensorineural hearing level from the brainstem evoked response. Archives of Otolaryngology 104: 456

Jerger J, Oliver T, Stach B 1985 Auditory brainstem response testing strategies. In: Jacobson J T (ed) The auditory brainstem response. College-Hill Press, San Diego, Calif., pp 372–388

Jewett D L, Williston J S 1971 Auditory-evoked far fields averaged from scalp of humans. Brain 94: 681–696

Jewett D L, Romano M N, Williston J S 1970 Human auditory evoked potentials. Possible brain-stem components detected on the scalp. Science 167: 1517–1518

Johnson E W 1979 Results of auditory tests in acoustic tumor patients (ch. 9). In: House W F, Luetje C M (eds) Acoustic tumors vol I: Diagnosis. University Park Press, Baltimore, Md.

Johnson J H, Kline D G 1978 Anterior inferior cerebellar artery aneurysms. Neurosurgery 48: 455–460

Joint Committee on Infant Hearing 1982 Position Statement. Paediatrics 60: 496–497

Jones J G, Heneghan C P H, Thornton C 1985 Functional assessment of the normal brain during general anaesthesia. In: Kaufman L (ed) Anaesthesia: Review 3. Churchill Livingstone, Edinburgh, pp 91–98

Josey A F, Glasscock M E, Jackson G 1984 Abnormal brainstem auditory evoked potentials in a neurotologic population. In: Nodar R H, Barber C (eds) Evoked potentials II. Butterworth, Boston, pp 224–227

Kaga K, Hink R F, Shinoda Y, Suzuki J 1980 Evidence of a primary cortical origin of middle latency auditory evoked responses during open-heart surgery with hypothermia. EEG Clinical Neurophysiology 55: 268

Kaga K, Tanaka Y 1980 Auditory brainstem response and behavioral audiometry: Developmental correlates. Archives of Otolaryngology 106: 564–566

Karnahl T, Benning C D 1972 Effect of sedation upon evoked response audiometry: Amplitude and latency versus sound pressure level. Archiv für Klinische und experimentelle Ohren-Nasen-und Kehlkopfheilkunde 201: 181–188

Kavanagh K T, Harker L A, Tyler R S 1984 Auditory brainstem and middle latency responses II: Threshold responses to a 500 Hz tone pip. Annals of Otology, Rhinology and Laryngology 93: 8–12

Keen M, Graham J M 1984 Clinical monitoring of the effect of gentamicin by electrocochleography. Journal of Laryngology and Otology 98: 11–21

Kemp D T 1978 Stimulated acoustic emissions from within the human auditory system. Journal of the Acoustical Society of America 64: 1386–1391

Kevanishvili Z, Aponchenko V 1979 Frequency composition of brainstem auditory evoked potentials. Scandinavian Audiology 8: 51–55

Kevanishvili Z, Aponchenko V 1981 Click polarity inversion effects upon the human brainstem auditory evoked potential. Scandinavian Audiology 10: 141–147

Khechinashvili S N, Kevanishvili Z S 1974 Experiences in computer audiometry (ECochG and ERA). Audiology 13: 391–402

Kiang N Y-S, Christ A H, French M A, Edwards A C 1963 Postauricular electric response to acoustic stimulation in humans. Lab Electronics MIT. Quarterly Progress Report on Research 68: 218–225

Kiang N Y-S, Watanabe T, Thomas E C et al 1965 Discharge patterns of single fibers in the cat's auditory nerve. Research monograph 35, MIT Press, Cambridge, Mass.

Kiang N Y S, Moxon E C, Kahn A R 1976 The relationships of gross cochlear potentials recorded from the cochlea to single unit activity in the auditory nerve. In: Ruben R J, Elberling C, Salomon G (eds) Electrocochleography. University Park Press, Baltimore, pp 95–115

Kileny P 1981 The frequency specificity of tone-pip evoked auditory brainstem responses. Ear and Hearing 2: 270–275

Kileny P, Dobson D, Gelfand E T 1983 Middle latency auditory evoked responses during open heart surgery with hypothermia. Electroencephalography and Clinical Neurophysiology 55: 268

Kileny P, Kemink J 1987 Electric MLRs in cochlear implant candidates. International Electric Response Audiometry Study Group x Biennial Symposium (Charlottesville, V.). ERA Newsletter 19: 186

Kileny P, McIntyre J W R 1985 The ABR in intraoperative monitoring. In: Jacobson J T (ed) The Auditory Brainstem Response. College-Hill Press, San Diego, Calif., pp 237–251

Kileny P, Shea S L 1986 Middle-latency and 40-Hz auditory evoked responses in normal-hearing subjects: Click and 500-Hz thresholds. Journal of Speech and Hearing Research 29: 20–28

King T T, Morrison A W 1980 Translabyrinthine and transtentorial removal of acoustic nerve tumours: Results of 150 cases. Journal of Neurosurgery 52: 210–216

Kingston J E, Abramovich S, Billings R J et al 1986 Assessment of the effect of chemotherapy and radiotherapy on the auditory function of children with cancer. Clinical Otolaryngology 11: 403–409

Knight R T, Hillyard S A, Woods D L et al 1980 The effects of frontal and temporal-parietal lesions in the auditory evoked potential in man. Electroencephalography and Clinical Neurophysiology 50: 112–124

Kodera K, Marsh R R, Suzuki M, Suzuki J 1983 Portions of tone pips contributing to frequency-selective auditory brain-stem responses. Audiology 22: 209–218

Kraus N, Ozdamar O, Hier D, Stein L 1982 Auditory middle latency responses (MLRs) in patients with cortical lesions. Electroencephalography and Clinical Neurophysiology 54: 275

Kumagami H, Nishida H, Baba M 1982 Electrocochleographic study of Ménière's disease. Archives of Otolaryngology 108: 284–288

Lader M, Norris H 1969 The effects of nitrous oxide on the human auditory evoked response. Psychopharmacologia (Berlin) 16: 115–127

Lang J 1981 Facial and vestibulocochlear nerve, topographic anatomy and variations. In: Samii M, Jannetta P J (eds) The cranial nerves. Springer, New York

Laukli E 1983 High-pass and notch noise masking in suprathreshold brainstem response audiometry. Scandinavian Audiology 12: 109–115

Laukli E, Mair I W S 1981 Early auditory-evoked responses: Filter effects. Audiology 20: 300–312

Lempert J, Meltzer P E, Wever E G, Lawrence M 1950 The cochleogram and its clinical applications. Concluding observations. Archives of Otolaryngology 51: 307–311

Lempert J, Wever E G, Lawrence M 1947 The cochleogram and its clinical applications: a preliminary report. Archives of Otolaryngology 45: 61–67

Lenarz T 1985 Treatment of tinnitus with lidocaine and tocainide. Scandinavian Audiology (suppl.) 26: 49–51

Lenarz T, Gulzow J, Grozinger M, Hoth S 1986 Clinical evaluation of 40-Hz middle-latency responses in adults: Frequency specific threshold estimation and suprathreshold amplitude characteristics. Journal of Oto-rhino-laryngology and its related specialties, Basel 48: 24–32

Lenarz T, Gulzow J, Zeuner H, Trost H 1987 CM, CAP and brain-stem auditory evoked potentials during systemic infusion of lidocaine, tocainide and phenytoin. International Electric Response Audiometry Study Group x Biennial Symposium (Charlottesville, V.). ERA Newsletter 19: 126

Lev A, Sohmer H 1972 Sources of averaged neural responses recorded in animal and human subjects during cochlear audiometry (electrocochleography). Archiv für Klinische und experimentelle Ohren-Nasen und Kehlkopfheilkunde 201: 79–90

Levin et al 1984 Annals of Otology, Rhinology and Laryngology 93: 117–120

Liberman M C 1982 Single neuron labeling in the cat auditory nerve. Science 216: 1239–1241

Lintchicum F H, Khalessi M M, Churchill D 1979 Electronystagmographic caloric bithermal vestibular test (ENG): Results in acoustic tumor cases. In: House W F, Luetje C M (eds) Acoustic tumors vol. I: Diagnosis. University Park Press, Baltimore, Md.

Lorente de Nó 1981 The primary acoustic nuclei. Raven Press, New York

Lynn G, Taylor P, Gilroy J 1980 Auditory evoked potentials in multiple sclerosis. Electroencephalography and Clinical Neurophysiology 50: 167

Maast T E 1965 Short latency human evoked responses to clicks. Journal of Applied Physiology 20: 725

McAlpine D, Lumsden C E, Acheson E D 1972 Multiple sclerosis – a reappraisal. Churchill Livingstone, Edinburgh

McCormick B, Curnock D A, Spavins F 1984 Auditory screening of special care neonates using the auditory response cradle. Archives of Disease in Childhood 59: 1168–1172

McFarland W H, Vivion M C, Goldstein R 1977 Middle components of the AER to tone pips in normal-hearing and hearing impaired subjects. Journal of Speech and Hearing Research 20: 781–798

McGee T J, Clemis J D 1982 Effects of conductive hearing loss on auditory brainstem response. Annals of Otology, Rhinology and Laryngology 91: 304–309

Marshall N K, Douchin E 1981 Circadian variation in the latency of brainstem responses: Its relation to body temperature. Science 212: 356–358

Martin J A M 1982 Aetiological factors relating to childhood deafness in the European Community. Audiology 21: 149–158

Mason S M, Adams W 1984 An automated microcomputer-based electric response audiometry system for machine scoring of auditory evoked potentials. Clinical Physical and Physiological Measurement 5: 219–222

Mason S M, Singh C B, Brown P M 1980 Assessment of non-invasive electrocochleography. Journal of Laryngology and Otology 94: 707–718

Mauguière F, Brechard S, Pernier J, Courjon J, Schott B 1982 Anosognosia with hemiplegia: Auditory evoked potential studies. In: Courjon J, Mauguière F, Revol M (eds) Clinical application of evoked potentials in neurology. Raven Press, New York, pp 271–278

Maurer K 1985 Uncertainties of topodiagnosis of auditory nerve and brain-stem evoked potentials due to rarefaction and condensation stimuli. Electroencephalography and Clinical Neurophysiology 62: 135–140

Maurer K, Schafer E, Leitner H 1980 The effect of varying stimulus polarity (rarefaction vs. condensation) on early auditory evoked potentials (EAEPs). Electroencephalography and Clinical Neurophysiology 50: 332–334

Maurizi M, Altissimi G, Ottaviani F, Paludetti G, Bambini M 1982 Auditory brainstem responses (ABR) in the aged. Scandinavian Audiology 11: 213–221

Maurizi M, Ottaviani F, Almadori G et al 1987 Auditory brainstem and middle-latency responses in Bell's palsy. Audiology 26: 111–116

Mendel M I 1974 Influence of stimulus level and sleep stage on the early components of the averaged electroencephalographic response to clicks during all-night sleep. Journal of Speech and Hearing Research 17: 5–17

Mendel M I, Goldstein R 1969 The effect of test conditions on the early components of the averaged electroencephalic response. Journal of Speech and Hearing Research 12: 344–350

Mendel M I, Goldstein R 1971 Early components of the averaged electroencephalic response to constant level clicks during all-night sleep. Journal of Speech and Hearing Research 14: 829–840

Mendel M I, Adkinson C D, Harker L A 1977 Middle components of the auditory evoked potentials in infants. Annals of Otology, Rhinology and Laryngology 86: 293–299

Meyerhoff W L 1981 The management of sudden sensorineural hearing loss. In: Paparella M, Meyerhoff W L (eds) Sensorineural hearing loss, vertigo and tinnitus. Ear Clinics International vol I. Williams and Wilkins, Baltimore, Md.

Mitchell C, Clemis J D 1977 Audiograms derived from the brainstem response. Laryngoscope 87: 2016–2022

Miyamoto R T, Brown D D 1987a Clinical applications of the electrically evoked brainstem response. In: Banfai P (ed) Cochlear implants: Current situation. International Cochlear Symposium 1987 (Duren, West Germany). Bermann, Erkelenz, pp 87–96

Miyamoto R T, Brown D D 1987b Electrically evoked brainstem responses in cochlear implant recipients. Otolaryngology – Head and Neck Surgery 96: 34–38

Moffat D A, Gibson W P R, Ramsden R T, Morrison A W, Booth J B 1978 Transtympanic electrocochleography in the diagnosis of retrocochlear tumours. Clinical Otolaryngology 1: 153–157

Moller A R 1983a Auditory physiology. Academic Press, New York

Moller A R 1983b On the origin of the compound action potentials (N1, N2) of the cochlea of the rat. Experimental Neurology 80: 633–644

Moller A R, Jannetta P J 1983a Interpretation of the brainstem auditory evoked potentials: Results from intracranial recordings in humans. Scandinavian Audiology (Stockholm) 12: 125–133

Moller A R, Jannetta P J 1983b Monitoring auditory functions during cranial nerve microvascular decompression operations by direct recording from the eighth nerve. Journal of Neurosurgery 59: 493–499

Moller A R, Jannetta P J 1985 Neural generators of the auditory brainstem response. In: Jacobson J T (ed) The auditory brainstem response. College-Hill Press, San Diego, Calif., pp 13–31

Moller A R, Jannetta P J, Moller M B 1982 Intracranially recorded auditory nerve response in man: New interpretations of BSER. Archives of Otolaryngology 108: 77–82

Moller M B, Moller A R (1989) Auditory brainstem evoked responses (ABR) in diagnosis of eighth nerve and brainstem lesions. In: Pinheiro M, Musiek F (eds) Assessment of central auditory dysfunction: its foundations and clinical correlates. Williams and Wilkins, Baltimore

Moller M B, Moller A R, Jannetta P J 1982 BSER in patients with hemifacial spasm. Laryngoscope 92: 848–852

Moore J K, Moore R Y 1971 A comparative study of the superior olivary complex in the primate brain. Folia Primatology (Basel) 16: 35–51

Morgan D E, Zimmerman M C, Dubno J R 1987 Auditory brainstem response characteristics in the full-term newborn infant. Annals of Otology, Rhinology and Laryngology 96: 142–151

Mori N, Asai H, Doi T, Matsunaga T 1987 Diagnostic value of extratympanic
electrocochleography in Ménière's disease. Audiology 26: 103–110

Mori N, Saeki K, Matsunaga T, Asai H 1982 Comparison between AP and SP parameters
in trans- and extratympanic electrocochleography. Audiology 21: 228–241

Morihisa J M, Duffy F H, Wyatt R J 1983 Brain electrical activity mapping (BEAM) in
schizophrenic patients. Archives of General Psychiatry 40/7: 719–728

Morrison A W 1975 Management of sensorineural deafness. Butterworth, London

Morrison A W, Gibson W P R, Beagley H A 1976 Transtympanic electrocochleography in
the diagnosis of retrocochlear tumours. Clinical Otolaryngology 1: 153–157

Morrison A W, Moffat D A, O'Connor A F 1980 Clinical usefulness of
electrocochleography in Ménière's disease: An analysis of dehydrating agents. The
Otological Clinics of North America 13: (4)703–721

Mouney D F, Berlin C I, Cullen J K et al 1978 Changes in human eighth nerve action
potential as a function of stimulation rate. Archives of Otolaryngology 104: 551–554

Musiek F E, Collegly K M 1985 ABR in eighth nerve and low brainstem lesions. In:
Jacobson J T (ed) The auditory brainstem response. College-Hill Press, San Diego,
Calif., 181–202

Musiek F E, Geurkink N A 1981 Auditory brainstem and middle latency evoked response
sensitivity near threshold. Annals of Otology, Rhinology and Laryngology 90: 236–240

Musiek F E, Geurkink N A, Spiegel P 1987 Audiologic and other clinical findings in a
case of basilar artery aneurism. Archives of Otolaryngology – Head and Neck Surgery
113: 772–776

Nedzelski J M, Tator C H 1980 Surgical management of cerebellopontine angle tumours.
Journal of Otolaryngology 9: 105–112

Nicol T, Chao-Charia K K 1981 Clinical anatomy of the ear. In: Beagley H A (ed)
Audiology and audiological medicine. vol I, p 33

Nodar R H, Hahn J F, Erenberg G, Rothner A D 1984 Improvement of brainstem
auditory evoked potential test results following intervention for brainstem tumors. In:
Nodar R H, Barber C (eds) Evoked potentials II (The Second International Evoked
Potential Symposium). Butterworth, Boston, Mass., pp 228–236

Northern J L, Downs M P 1984 Hearing in children. 3rd edn. Williams and Wilkins,
Baltimore, Md.

Ohashi T, Yoshie N, Shimada K 1985 Clinical application of summating potentials in the
diagnosis of inner ear diseases. In: Myers E G (ed) New dimensions in
otorhinolaryngology – head and neck surgery. vol 2. Excerpta Medica, Amsterdam,
pp 111–114

Okitsu T 1984 Middle components of the auditory evoked response in young children.
Scandinavian Audiology 13: 83

Ozdamar O, Kraus N 1983 Auditory middle-latency responses in humans. Audiology
22: 34–49

Ozdamar O, Kraus N, Curry F 1982 Auditory brainstem and middle latency responses in a
patient with cortical deafness. Electroencephalography and Clinical Neurophysiology
53: 224–230

Pantev Ch, Lutkenhoner B, Hoke M, Hehnerpz K 1986 Comparison between
simultaneously recorded audiometry – evoked magnetic fields and potentials elicited by
ipsilateral, contralateral and binaural toneburst stimulation. Audiology 25: 54–61

Papanicolaou A C, Loring D W, Raz N, Eisenberg H M 1985 Relationship between
stimulus intensity and the P300. Psychophysiology 22: 326

Paparella M 1985 The cause (multifactorial inheritance) and pathogenesis (endolymphatic
malabsorption) of Ménière's disease and its symptoms (mechanical and chemical). Acta
Otolaryngologica 99: 445–451

Paradise J L 1982 Editorial retrospective: Tympanometry. New England Journal of
Medicine 307: 1074–1076

Parker D J, Thornton A R D 1978a Cochlear travelling wave velocities calculated from the
derived components of the cochlear nerve and brainstem evoked responses of the human
auditory system. Scandinavian Audiology 7: 67–70

Parker D J, Thornton A R D 1978b Derived cochlear nerve and brainstem evoked
responses of the human auditory system: The effect of masking and derived band.
Scandinavian Audiology 7: 73–80

Parker D J, Thornton A R D 1978c The validity of the derived cochlear nerve and brainstem evoked responses of the human auditory system. Scandinavian Audiology 7: 45–52

Parving A, Salomon G, Elberling C, Larsen B, Lassen N A 1980 Middle components of the auditory evoked response in bilateral temporal lobe lesions. Scandinavian Audiology 9: 161

Peters J G 1986 An automated infant screener using advanced evoked response technology. Hearing Journal 39(9): 25–30

Pickles J O 1985 Hearing and listening. In: Swash M, Kennard C (eds) Scientific basis of clinical neurology. Churchill Livingstone, Edinburgh, pp 188–200

Pickles J O 1982 An introduction to the physiology of hearing. Academic Press, New York

Pickles J O 1985 The physiology of the cochlea. In: Gray R F (ed) Cochlear implants. Croom Helm, London, pp 27–32

Pickles J O, Comis S D, Osborn M P 1984 Cross-links between stereocilia in the guinea-pig organ of Corti, and their possible relation to sensory transduction. Hearing Research 15: 103–112

Picton T W, Hillyard S A, Galambos R 1976 Habituation and attention in the auditory system. In: Keidel W D, Neff W D (eds) Handbook of sensory physiology vol 5, no 3. Springer, New York

Picton T W, Hillyard S A, Kraus H J, Galambos R 1974 Human auditory evoked potentials: Evaluation components. Electroencephalography and Clinical Neurophysiology 36: 179–190

Picton T W, Oullette J, Hamel G, Smith A D 1979 Brainstem evoked potentials to tone pips in notched noise. Journal of Otolaryngology 8: 289–314

Picton T W, Stapells D R, Campbell K B 1981 Auditory evoked potentials from the human cochlea and brainstem. Journal of Otolaryngology (suppl. 9) 10: 1–41

Picton T W, Stuss D T, Champagne S C, Nelson R F 1984 The effects of age on human event-related potentials. Psychophysiology 21: 312

Pijl S 1987 Effects of click polarity on ABR peak latency and morphology in a clinical population. Journal of Otolaryngology 16: 89–96

Portmann M, Aran J-M 1971 Electro-cochleography. Laryngoscope 81: 899–910

Portmann M, Aran J-M, Le Bert G 1968 Acta Otolaryngologica (Stockholm) 65: 105

Portmann M, Cazals Y, Negrevergne M, Aran J-M 1980 Transtympanic and surface recordings in the diagnosis of retrocochlear disorders. Acta Otolaryngologica 89: 362–369

Prasher D K, Gibson W P R 1980 Brainstem auditory evoked potentials: A comparative study of monaural versus binaural stimulation in the detection of MS. Electroencephalography and Clinical Neurophysiology 50: 247–253

Prasher D K, Gibson W P R 1983 Brainstem auditory evoked potentials and electrocochleography: Comparison of different criteria for the detection of acoustic neuroma and other cerebello-pontine angle tumours. British Journal of Audiology 17: 163–174

Pratt H, Ben-David Y, Peled R, Podoshin L, Scharf B 1981 Auditory brainstem evoked potentials: Clinical promise of increasing stimulus rate. Electroencephalography and Clinical Neurophysiology 51: 80–90

Pratt H, Ben-Yitzhak E, Attias J 1984 Auditory brainstem potentials evoked by clicks in notch-filtered masking noise: Audiological relevance. Audiology 23: 380–397

Pratt H, Harel Z, Friedman Y, Golos E 1984 Voltage-space analysis of short-latency evoked potentials. In: Nodar R H, Barber C (eds) Evoked potentials II. Butterworth, Boston, Mass., pp 90–95

Pratt H, Sohmer H 1976 Intensity and rate functions of cochlear and brainstem evoked responses to click stimulation in man. Archives of Otolaryngology 212: 85–92

Quaranta A, Mininni F, Longo G 1986 ABR in multiple sclerosis – ipsi-versus contralateral derivation. Scandinavian Audiology 15: 125–128

Ragazzoni A, Amantine A, Rossi L et al 1982 Brainstem auditory evoked potentials and vertebrobasilar reversible ischaemic attacks. Advances in Neurology 2: 187–194

Ramsden R T, Latif A, O'Malley S 1985 Electrocochleographic changes in acute salicylate overdosage. Journal of Laryngology and Otology 99: 1269–1273

Ramsden R T, Wilson P, Gibson W P 1980 Immediate effects of intravenous tobramycin and gentamicin on human cochlear function. Journal of Laryngology and Otology 94: 521–528

Rasmussen G L 1942 An efferent cochlear bundle. Anatatomical Record 82: 441

Reid A, Thornton A R D 1983 The effects of contralateral masking upon brainstem electric responses. British Journal of Audiology 17: 155–162

Rhys Evans P H, Comis S D, Osborn M P, Pickles J O, Jeffries J R 1985 Cross-links between stereocilia in the human organ of Corti. Journal of Laryngology and Otology 99: 11–19

Robinson K H, Rudge P 1975 Auditory evoked responses in multiple sclerosis. Lancet (May) 24: 1164–1166

Robinson K H, Rudge P 1977 Abnormalities of the auditory evoked potential in patients with multiple sclerosis. Brain 100: 19–49

Robinson K H, Rudge P 1980 The use of the auditory evoked potential in the diagnosis of multiple sclerosis. Journal of Neurological Science 45: 235–244

Robinson K H, Rudge P 1981 Centrally generated auditory potentials. In: Halliday A M (ed) Evoked potentials in clinical testing. Churchill Livingstone, Edinburgh, pp 345–372

Robinson K H, Rudge P 1983 The differential diagnosis of cerebello-pontine angle lesions. Journal of the Neurological Sciences 60: 1–21

Robles L, Ruggero M, Rich N 1986 Mossbauer measurements of the mechanical response to single-tone and two-tone stimuli at the base of the chinchilla cochlea. In: Allen J B, Hall J L, Hubbard A, Neely S T, Tubis A (eds) Peripheral auditory mechanisms. Springer, Berlin

Ronis B J 1966 Cochlear potentials in otosclerosis. Laryngoscope 73: 212–231

Rosenblatt B, Majnemer A 1984 Brainstem auditory evoked potentials in children with brainstem encephalitis. In: Nodar R H, Barber C (eds) Evoked potentials II. Butterworth, Boston, Mass., pp 216–223

Rosenhall U, Hedner M, Bjorkman G 1981 ABR and brainstem lesions. Scandinavian Audiology (suppl. 13): 117–123

Rosenhamer H J 1977 Observations on electrical brainstem responses in retrocochlear hearing loss. Scandinavian Audiology 6: 179–196

Rosenhamer H J 1981a The auditory evoked brainstem electric response (ABR) in cochlear hearing loss. Scandinavian Audiology (suppl. 13): pp 83–93

Rosenhamer H J 1981b Brainstem changes in chronic alcoholism revealed by ABR. Scandinavian Audiology (suppl. 13): 133–134

Rosenhamer H J, Lindstrom B, Lundborg J 1980 On the use of click evoked electric brainstem responses in audiological diagnosis II: The influence of sex and age upon the normal response. Scandinavian Audiology 9: 93–100

Rothera M, Conway M, Brightwell A, Graham J 1986 Evaluation of patients for cochlear implant by promontory stimulation. British Journal of Audiology 20: 25–28

Rotteveel J J, Colon E J, de Graaf R, Notermans S L H, Stoelinga G B A, Visco Y 1986 The central auditory conduction at term date and three months after birth III: Middle latency responses (MLRs). Scandinavian Audiology 15: 75–84

Rotteveel J J, Colon E J, Notermans S L H, Stoelinga G B A, de Graaf R, Visco Y 1986 The central auditory conduction at term date and three months after birth IV: Auditory cortical responses. Scandinavian Audiology 15: 85–95

Rowe M J 1978 Normal variability of the brainstem auditory evoked responses in young and old adult subjects. Electroencephalography and Clinical Neurophysiology 44: 459–470

Ruben R J 1967 Cochlear potentials as a diagnostic test in deafness. In: Graham A B (ed) Sensorineural hearing processes and disorders. Little, Brown, Boston, Mass.

Ruben R J, Bordley J E, Lieberman A T 1961 Cochlear potentials in man. Laryngoscope 71: 1141–1164

Ruben R J, Hudson W, Chiong A 1982 Anatomical and physiological effects of chronic section of the eighth nerve in the cat. Acta Otolaryngologica (Stockholm) 55: 473–484

Ruben R J, Knickerbocker G G, Sekula J et al 1959 Cochlear microphonics in man: A preliminary report. Laryngoscope 69: 665–671

Ruben R J, Lieberman A T, Bordley J E 1962 Some observations on cochlear potentials and nerve action potentials in children. Laryngoscope 72: 545–554

Rudge P 1983 Clinical neuro-otology. Churchill Livingstone, Edinburgh, pp 187–216

Russell I J, Sellick P M 1978 Intracellular studies of hair cells in the mammalian cochlea. Journal of Physiology (London) 284: 261–290

Ruth R A, Hildenbrand D L, Cantrell R W 1982 A study of methods used to enhance wave I in the auditory brainstem response. Otolaryngology and Head and Neck Surgery 90: 635–640

Ryerson S G, Beagley H A 1981 Brainstem electric response and electrocochleography: A comparison of threshold sensitivities in children. British Journal of Audiology 15: 41–48

Sabin H I, Bentivoglio P, Symon L, Cheesman A D, Prasher D, Momma F 1987 Intra-operative electrocochleography to monitor cochlear potentials during acoustic neuroma excision. Acta Neurochirurgica 85: 110–116

Salamy A, Fenn C B, Bronshvag M 1979 Ontogenesis of human brainstem evoked potential amplitude. Developmental Psychobiology 12: 519–526

Salamy A, McKean C M 1976 Postnatal development of the human brainstem potentials during the first year of life. Electroencephalography and Clinical Neurophysiology 40: 418–426

Salamy A, Mendelson T, Tooley W H 1982 Developmental profiles for the brainstem auditory evoked potential. Early Human Development 6: 331–339

Salomon G, Elberling C 1971 Cochlear nerve potentials recorded from the ear canal in man. Acta Otolaryngologica (Stockholm) 71: 4–15

Salt A N 1982 presentation on ear canal probe microphone measurements of click polarity. 1st International Conference on Standards for Auditory Brainstem Response Measurement. Laguna Beach, Calif.

Salt A N, Thornton A R D 1984 The choice of stimulus polarity for brainstem auditory evoked potentials in the clinic. In: Nodar R H, Barber C (eds) Evoked potentials II. Butterworth, Boston, Mass., pp 203–215

Sand T, Sulg I 1984 Influence of click phase and rate upon latencies and latency distributions of the normal brainstem auditory evoked potentials. Electrocochleography and Clinical Neurophysiology 57: 561–570

Sanders R, Durieux-Smith A, Hyde M L, Kileny P, Jacobson J T, Murnane O 1985 Incidence of hearing loss in high-risk and intensive care nursery infants. Journal of Otolaryngology (suppl. 14) 14: 28–33

Saunders J W, Josey A F, Glasscock M E 1974 Audiologic evaluation in cochlear and eighth nerve disorders. Archives of Otolaryngology 100: 283–289

Saunders J G, Schneider M E, Dear S P 1985 The structure and function of actin in the hair cells. Journal of the Acoustic Society of America 78: 299–311

Scherg M, von Cramon D 1985 A new interpretation of the generators of BAEP waves I–V: Results of a spatio-temporal dipole model. Electroencephalography and Clinical Neurophysiology 62: 290–299

Schimmel H 1967 The [±] reference: accuracy of estimated mean components in average response studies. Science 157: 92–93

Schuknecht H F 1974 Pathology of the ear. Harvard University Press, Cambridge, Mass.

Schuknecht H F 1981 Ear disease and hearing loss: Where do we go from here? In: Paparella M, Meyerhoff W L (eds) Sensorineural hearing loss, vertigo and tinnitus. Ear Clinics international, vol I. Williams and Wilkins, Baltimore, Md.

Schuknecht H F, Gulya A J 1983 Endolymphatic hydrops – an overview of classification. Annals of Otology, Rhinology and Laryngology (suppl.) 106: 1–20

Schwartz D M, Berry G A 1985 Normative aspects of the ABR. In: Jacobson J T (ed) The auditory brainstem response. College-Hill Press, San Diego, Calif., pp 65–97

Sklare D A, Lynn G E 1984 P3 event-related potential: Normative aspects and within-subject variability. Electroencephalography and Clinical Neurophysiology 59: 420–424

Sellick P M, Patuzzi R, Johnston B M 1982 Measurement of basilar membrane motion in the guinea pig using the Mossbauer technique. Journal of the Acoustic Society of America 72: 131–141

Sellick P M, Russell I L 1978 Intracellular studies of cochlear hair cells. In: Naunton R F, Fernandez C (eds) Evoked electrical activity in the auditory nervous system. Academic Press, New York

Selters W A, Brackmann D E 1977 Acoustic tumor detection with brainstem electrical response audiometry. Archives of Otolaryngology 103: 181–187

Selters W A, Brackmann D E 1979 Brainstem electrical response audiometry in tumour detection. In: House W F, Luetje C M (eds) Acoustic tumors. vol I. University Park Press, Baltimore, Md.

Shah S N, Bhargava V K, McKean C M 1978 Maturational changes in early auditory evoked potentials and myelination of the inferior colliculus in rats. Neuroscience 3: 561–563

Shaia F, Sheehy J 1976 Sudden sensorineural hearing impairment: A report of 1220 cases. Laryngoscope 86: 389–398

Shallop J K, Osterhammel P A 1983 A comparative study of measurements of SN-10 and 40/s middle latency responses in newborns. Scandinavian Audiology 12: 91–95

Shallop J K, Osterhammel P A, Tubergen L B 1984 Comparative measurements of SN10 and the 40/s middle-latency response in newborns. In: Nodar R H, Barber C (eds) Evoked potentials II. Butterworth, Boston, Mass., pp 548–552

Shanon E, Gould S, Himelfarb M Z 1981 Assessment of functional integrity of brainstem auditory pathways by stimulus stress. Audiology 20: 65–71

Shanon E, Himelfarb M, Zikk D 1985 Measurement of auditory brainstem potentials in Bell's palsy. Laryngoscope 95: 206–209

Sheehy J L 1979 Neuro-otological evaluation. In: House W F, Luetje C M (eds) Acoustic tumors, vol I: Diagnosis. University Park Press, Baltimore, Md.

Simmons F B 1976 Clinical evaluation of hearing loss. In: Ruben R J, Elberling C, Salomon G (eds) Electrocochleography. University Park Press, Baltimore, Md., pp 89–93

Simmons F B 1980 Patterns of deafness in newborns. Laryngoscope 90: 448–453

Simmons F B, Luster H S, Myers T, Shelton C 1987 Electrically induced auditory brainstem response as a clinical tool in estimating nerve survival. Annals of Otology, Rhinology and Laryngology (suppl. 128) 92: 96

Simson R, Vaughan H G, Ritter W The scalp topography of potentials in auditory and visual go/no go tasks. Electroencephalography and Clinical Neurophysiology 43: 864–875

Singh C B, Mason S M, Brown P M 1980 Extratympanic electrocochleography in clinical use. In: Barber C (ed) Evoked potentials. MTP Press, Lancaster, pp 357–366

Sklare D A, Lynn G E 1984 Latency of the P3 event-related potential: Normative aspects and within-subject variability. Electroencephalography and Clinical Neurophysiology 59: 420–424

Smith L, Simmons F B 1983 Estimating eighth nerve survival by electrical stimulation. Annals of Otology, Rhinology and Laryngology 92: 19–23

Smith R L 1979 Adaptation, saturation, and physiological masking in single auditory-nerve fibers. Journal of the Acoustic Society of America 65: 166–178

Smyth G D, Gordon D S, Campbell R, Kerr A G 1982 The facial nerve in acoustic neuroma surgery. Journal of Laryngology and Otology 96: 335–346

Sohmer H, Feinmesser M 1967 Cochlear action potentials recorded from the external ear in man. Annals of Otology, Rhinology and Laryngology 76: 427–435

Sohmer H, Feinmesser M 1973 Routine use of electrocochleography (cochlear audiometry) in human subjects. Audiology 12: 167–173

Soucek S 1989 A study of hearing in the elderly using non-invasive electrocochleography and auditory brainstem response. Journal of Otolaryngology 16: 345–353

Spoendlin H 1985 Inner ear. In: Beagley H A (ed) Audiology and audiological medicine. Oxford University Press, Oxford, vol 1, pp 33

Spoendlin H 1986 Receptoneural and innervation aspects of the inner ear anatomy with respect to cochlear mechanics. Scandinavian Audiology (suppl.) 25: 27–34

Spoor A, Eggermont J J, Odenthal D W 1976 Comparison of human and animal data concerning adaptation and masking of eighth nerve compound action potential. In: Ruben R J, Elberling C, Salomon G (eds) Electrocochleography. University Park Press, Baltimore, Md., pp 183–198

Staewehn W S, Allison D, Harris K et al 1980 Determining acoustic condensation and rarefaction of earphones for brainstem auditory evoked responses. American Journal of EEG Technology 20: 133–138

Stapells D R, Picton T W 1981 Technical aspects of brainstem evoked potential audiometry using tones. Ear and Hearing 2: 20–29

Stapells D R, Picton T W, Perez-Abalo M, Read D, Smith A 1985 Frequency specificity in evoked potential audiometry. In: Jacobson J T (ed) The auditory brainstem response. College-Hill Press, San Diego, Calif., pp 147–177

Starr A, Achor L J 1975 Auditory brainstem responses in neurological disease. Archives of Neurology 32: 761–768

Starr A, Amlie R N, Martin W H, Sanders S 1977 Development of auditory function in newborn infants revealed by auditory brainstem potentials. Paediatrics 60: 831–839

Starr A, Hamilton A E 1976 Correlation between confirmed sites of neurological lesions and abnormalities of far-field auditory brainstem responses. Electroencephalography and Clinical Neurophysiology 41: 595–608

Starr A, Rosenberg C, Don M, Davis H (eds) 1984 Proceedings of the international conference on standards for auditory brainstem responses (ABR) testing. Sensory evoked potentials, Nearlands: CRS Amplifon

Stein L, Clark S, Krans N 1983 The hearing impaired infant: Patterns of identification and habilitation. Ear and Hearing 4: 232–236

Stein L, Ozdamar O, Schnabel M 1981 Auditory brainstem responses (ABR) with suspected deaf-blind children. Ear and Hearing 1: 30–40

Stelmasiak M 1954 Icones anatomicae encephali et medullae spinalis. Apud Medicorum Librorum Editores, Varsoviae, p 215

Stockard J E, Stockard J J, Westmoreland B F, Corfits J L 1979 Brainstem auditory-evoked responses. Normal variation as a function of stimulus and subject characteristics. Archives of Neurology 36: 823–831

Stockard J E, Stockard J J 1983 Recording and analyzing. In: Moore E J (ed) Bases of auditory brain-stem evoked responses. Grune & Stratton, New York, pp 255–286

Stockard J J, Sharbrough F W, Tinker J A 1978 Effects of hypothermia on the human brainstem auditory response. Annals of Neurology 3: 368–370

Stockard J J, Stockard J E, Sharbrough F W 1978 Nonpathologic factors influencing brainstem auditory evoked potentials. American Journal of Electroencephalography and Technology 18: 177–209

Stypulkovski P H, van den Honert C, Kvistad S, Muchow D 1985 Electrically evoked auditory brainstem responses: Experimental and clinical results. In: Lim D J (ed) Abstracts of the Eighth Midwinter Research Meeting: Association for Research in Otolaryngology. Clearwater, Fla., pp 106–107

Sutton S 1979 P300 – thirteen years later. In: Begleiter H (ed) Evoked potentials and behavior. Plenum Press, New York

Sutton S, Braren M, Zubin J, John E R 1965 Evoked potential correlates of stimulus uncertainty. Science 150: 1187–1188

Suzuki T, Hirabayashi M 1987 Age related morphological changes in auditory middle-latency response. Audiology 26: 312–320

Suzuki T, Horinchi K 1977 Effect of high-pass filter on auditory brainstem responses to tone pips. Scandinavian Audiology 6: 123–126

Tease D C, Eldridge D H, Davis H 1962 Cochlear responses to acoustic transients. An interpretation of whole nerve action potentials. Journal of the Acoustic Society of America 34: 1438–1489

Terkildsen K, Osterhammel P, Huis in't Veld F 1973 Far-field electrocochleography electrode positions. Scandinavian Audiology 2: 141–148

Terkildsen K, Osterhammel P, Huis in't Veld F 1974 Far-field electrocochleography, electrode positions. Scandinavian Audiology 4: 123–129

Terkildsen K, Osterhammel P, Huis in't Veld F 1975 Far-field electrocochleography. Frequency specificity of the response. Scandinavian Audiology 4: 167–172

Terkildsen K, Osterhammel P, Thomsen J 1981 The ABR and MLR in patients with acoustic neuromas. Scandinavian Audiology (suppl. 13): 103–108

Tilney L G, Saunders J C 1983 Actin filaments, stereocilia, and hair cells of the bird cochlea I: Length, number, width, and distribution of stereocilia of each hair cell are related to the position of the hair cell on the cochlea. Journal of Cell Biology 96: 807–821

Thornton A R D 1975 The use of post-auricular muscle responses. Journal of Laryngology and Otology 89: 997–1010

Thornton A R D 1983 Standardisation in evoked response measurements. British Journal of Audiology 17: 115–116

Thornton A R D 1984 Instrumentation for ABR recording. In: Starr A, Rosenberg C, Don M, Davis H (eds) Sensory evoked potentials I: An international conference on standards for auditory brainstem response (ABR) testing. CRS Amplifon, Milan pp 153–161

Thornton A R D 1986 Estimation of the number of patients who might be suitable for cochlear implant and similar procedures. British Journal of Audiology 20: 221–229

Thornton A R D 1987 Stimulus, recording and subject factors influencing ABR diagnostic criteria. British Journal of Audiology 21: 183–189

Thornton A R D 1987 Computers in audiology. In: Stephens S D G (ed) Scott-Brown's otolaryngology – adult audiology. Butterworth, London, pp 68–89

Thornton A R D, Farrell G 1989 Apparent travelling wave velocity changes in cases of endolymphatic hydrops. Scandinavian Audiology (in press)

Thornton A R D, Farrell G, Phillips A J, Haacke N P, Rhys-Williams S 1990 Verification of a new objective test of endolymphatic hydrops. Journal of Laryngology and Otology

Thornton A R D, Farrell G, Reid A, Peter S J 1990 Isochronic mapping; a preliminary report of a new technique. British Journal of Audiology (in press)

Thornton A R D, Ghariani A T 1989 (personal communication)

Thornton A R D, Hawkes C H 1976 Neurological applications of surface-recorded electrocochleography. Journal of Neurology, Neurosurgery and Psychiatry 39: 586–592

Thornton A R D, Yardley L, Farrell G 1987 The objective estimation of loudness discomfort level using auditory brainstem evoked responses. Scandinavian Audiology 16: 219–225

Thornton C, Heneghan C P H, James M F M, Jones J G 1984 The effects of halothane and enflurane on early auditory evoked potentials in humans. In: Nodar R H, Barber C (eds) Evoked potentials II. Butterworth, Boston, Mass., pp 483–490

Tjernstrom O, Casselbrant M 1981 Pressure chamber treatment in acute attacks of Ménière's disease. In: Vosteen K H et al (eds) Ménière's disease. Georg Thieme, Stuttgart, pp 211–214

Tonndorf J 1960 Shearing motion in scala media of cochlear models. Journal of the Acoustic Society of America 32: 238–244

Tonndorf J, Khanna S M 1976 Mechanics of the auditory system. In: Hinchcliffe R, Harrison D (eds) Scientific foundations of otolaryngology. William Heinemann, London, pp 237–252

Tsubokawa T, Nishimoto H, Yamamoto T, Kitamura M, Kitamaya Y, Morigasu N 1980 Assessment of brainstem damage by the brainstem auditory response in acute severe head injury. Journal of Neurology, Neurosurgery and Psychiatry 43: 1005–1011

Uri N, Schuchman J, Pratt H 1984 Auditory brainstem evoked potentials in Bell's palsy. Archives of Otolaryngology 110: 301–304

Walter W G 1964 Slow potential waves in the human brain associated with expectancy. Archives of Psychiatry 206: 309–322

Walter W G, Cooper R, Aldridge V J et al 1964 Contingent negative variation: An electric sign of sensory-motor association and expectancy in the human brain. Nature 203: 380–384

Waring M, Mikami K, Brimacombe J 1987 Changes in ABR stimuli in induction coil implant patients I: Effects of electrode stabilisation on stimulus current. International Electric Response Audiometry Study Group X Biennial Symposium. (Charlottesville, Va.) ERA Newsletter 19: 189

Warr W B 1978 The olivocochlear bundle : its origins and terminations in the cat. In: Naunton R F, Fernandez C (eds) Evoked electrical activity in the auditory nervous system. Academic Press, New York pp 43–65

Weiss C 1983 Use of behavioural tests in early diagnosis of hearing loss. Acta Otolaryngologica (suppl.)

Wever E G, Bray C W 1930 Auditory nerve impulses. Science 71: 215

Whitfield I C, Ross H F 1965 Cochlear microphonic and summating potentials and the outputs of individual hair cell generators. Journal of Acoustic Society of America 38: 126–131

Williston J S, Jewett D L, Martin W H 1981 Planar curve analysis of three-channel auditory brainstem response: A preliminary report. Brain Research 223: 181–184

Wolf K-E, Goldstein R 1978 Middle components AERs to tonal stimuli from normal neonates. Archives of otolaryngology 104: 508–513

Wolpaw J R, Penry J K 1977 Hemispheric differences in the auditory evoked response. Electroencephalography and Clinical Neurophysiology 43: 99–102

Wong P J H, Bickford R G 1980 Brainstem auditory evoked potentials: the use of noise estimate. Electroencephalopathy and Clinical Neurophysiology 50: 25–34

Woods D L, Clayworth C C 1985 Click spatial position influences and middle latency auditory evoked potentials (MAEPs) in humans. Electroencephalography and Clinical Neurophysiology 60: 122–129

World Health Organization 1967 The early detection and treatment of handicapping effect in young children. WHO, Copenhagen

Worthington D W, Peters J F 1980 Electrophysiologic audiometry. Annals of Otology, Rhinology and Laryngology 74: 59–62

Worthington D W, Peters J F 1980 Quantifiable hearing and no ABR: Paradox or error? Ear and Hearing 1: 281–285

Wright A 1984 Dimensions of cochlear stereocilia in man and the guinea pig. Hearing Research 13: 89–98

Yamada O, Kodera K, Yagi T 1979 Cochlear processes affecting wave V latency of the auditory evoked brainstem response. Scandinavian Audiology 8: 67–70

Yokoyama T, Ryu H, Uemura K, Miyamaoto T, Imamura Y 1987 Study of the constant wave form of ML-AEP in humans. Electroencephalography and Clinical Neurophysiology 67: 372–378

Yoshie N 1971 Clinical cochlear response audiometry by means of an average response computer. Non-surgical technique and clinical use. Revue de Laryngologie, Otologie, Rhinologie (Bordeaux) 92: 646–672

Yoshie N 1973 Diagnostic significance of the electrocochleogram in clinical audiometry. Audiology 12: 504–539

Yoshie N 1985 Clinical assessment of cochlear function by electrocochleography. In: Myers E (ed) New dimensions in otolaryngology – head and neck surgery. Excerpta Medica, Amsterdam, vol 1, pp 170–173

Yoshie N, Ohashi T, Suzuki T 1967 Non-surgical recording of auditory nerve action potentials in man. Laryngoscope 77: 76–85

Yoshie N, Okudaira T 1969 Acta Otolaryngologica (suppl.) 252: 89

Zanten G A van, Brocaar M P 1984 Frequency specific auditory brainstem responses to clicks masked by notched noise. Audiology 23: 253–364

Zerlin S, Nauton R F 1976 Effects of high-pass masking on the whole-nerve response to third octave audiometric clicks. In: Ruben R J, Elberling C, Salomon G (eds) Electrocochleography. University Park Press, Baltimore, Md., pp 207–213

Zulch K 1957 Brain tumors: Their biology and pathology. Springer, New York

Zwislocki J 1965 Analysis of some auditory characteristics. In: Bush R R, Luce R D, Galanter E (eds) Handbook of mathematical psychology. John Wiley, New York, vol 3, pp 1–97

Zwislocki J 1975 The role of the external and middle ear in sound transmission. In: Eagles E L (ed) The nervous system: Human communication and its disorders. Raven Press, New York, vol 3, 45–55

Zwislocki J 1985 Cochlear function – an analysis. Acta Otolaryngologica 100: 201–209

Index

235